BRISTOL-MYERS SQUIBB CANCER SYMPOSIA

Series Editor
STEPHEN K. CARTER*
Science and Technology Group
Bristol-Myers Squibb Company

1. Harris Busch, Stanley T. Crooke, and Yerach Daskal (Editors).
   Effects of Drugs on the Cell Nucleus, 1979.
2. Alan C. Sartorelli, John S. Lazo, and Joseph R. Bertino (Editors).
   Molecular Actions and Targets for Cancer Chemotherapeutic Agents, 1981.
3. Saul A. Rosenberg and Henry S. Kaplan (Editors).
   Malignant Lymphomas: Etiology, Immunology, Pathology, Treatment, 1982.
4. Albert H. Owens, Jr., Donald S. Coffey, and Stephen B. Baylin (Editors).
   Tumor Cell Heterogeneity: Origins and Implications, 1982.
5. Janet D. Rowley and John E. Ultmann (Editors).
   Chromosomes and Cancer: From Molecules to Man, 1983.
6. Umberto Veronesi and Gianni Bonadonna (Editors).
   Clinical Trials in Cancer Medicine: Past Achievements and Future Prospects, 1985.
7. Paul A. Marks (Editor).
   Genetics, Cell Differentiation, and Cancer, 1985.
8. Kenneth R. Harrap and Thomas A. Connors (Editors).
   New Avenues in Developmental Cancer Chemotherapy, 1987.
9. Paul V. Woolley III and Kenneth D. Tew (Editors).
   Mechanisms of Drug Resistance in Neoplastic Cells, 1988.

List continues at the end of this volume.

*Series Editor for Volumes 1–8 was Maxwell Gordon.

NUCLEAR PROCESSES AND ONCOGENES

Edited by

PHILLIP A. SHARP
Massachusetts Institute of Technology
Cambridge, Massachusetts

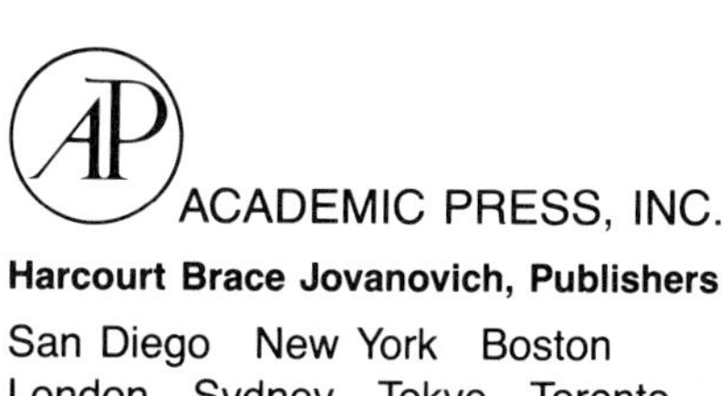

ACADEMIC PRESS, INC.
Harcourt Brace Jovanovich, Publishers
San Diego New York Boston
London Sydney Tokyo Toronto

This book is printed on acid-free paper. 

Academic Press, Inc.
1250 Sixth Avenue, San Diego, California 92101

United Kingdom Edition published by
Academic Press Limited
24–28 Oval Road, London NW1 7DX

Library of Congress Cataloging-in-Publication Data

Nuclear processes and oncogenes / edited by Phillip A. Sharp.
p. cm. -- (Bristol-Myers Squibb cancer symposia ; v. 14)
Based on the 14th Bristol-Myers Squibb Symposia on Cancer Research, held on Sept. 24–25, 1990 at Massachusetts Institute of Technology.
Includes bibliographical references and index.
ISBN 0-12-639025-8
1. Oncogenes--Congresses. 2. Antiocogenes--Congresses. 3. Gene expression--Congresses. 4. Genetic transcription--Regulation--Congresses. I. Sharp, Phillip A. II. Bristol-Myers Squibb Symposium on Cancer Research (14th : 1990 : Massachusetts Institute of Technology) III. Series.
[DNLM: 1. Cell Transformation, Neoplastic--congresses. 2. Gene Expression Regulation--congresses. 3. Neoplasms--genetics--congresses. 4. Nuclear Proteins--genetics--congresses. 5. Oncogenes--congresses. 6. Signal Transduction--congresses. QZ 202 N965 1990]
RC268.42.N84 1992
616.99'2042--dc20
DNLM/DLC
for Library of Congress 91-41218
CIP

PRINTED IN THE UNITED STATES OF AMERICA

92 93 94 95 96 97 BB 9 8 7 6 5 4 3 2 1

Contents

3 Transcriptional Regulation by Fos and Jun

TOM CURRAN, CORY ABATE, and PASCALE MACGREGOR

4 Independent Modulation of Differentiation and Proliferation in Erythroid Progenitors

HARTMUT BEUG, GABI DOEDERLEIN, and MARTIN ZENKE

PART II NUCLEAR TUMOR-SUPRESSOR GENES

5 The p53 Gene and Gene Product

ROBIN S. QUARTIN, CATHY A. FINLAY, and ARNOLD J. LEVINE

PART III REGULATION OF TRANSCRIPTION

Contributors

Numbers in parentheses indicate the pages on which the authors' contributions begin.

CORY ABATE (23), Roche Institute of Molecular Biology, Roche Research Center, Nutley, New Jersey 07110

SUZANNE J. BAKER (105), Oncology Center, Johns Hopkins University School of Medicine, Baltimore, Maryland 21231

MARISSA S. BARTOLOMEI (187), Department of Molecular Biology, Princeton University, Princeton, New Jersey 08544

HARTMUT BEUG (53), Institute of Molecular Pathology, A 1030 Vienna, Austria

J. MICHAEL BISHOP (11), Departments of Microbiology and Immunology, and Biochemistry and Biophysics, and the G. W. Hooper Research Foundation, University of California, San Francisco, San Francisco, California 94143

CAMILYNN I. BRANNAN (187), NCI–FCRDC (National Cancer Institute–Fredrick Cancer Research & Development Center), ABL-Basic Research Program, Fredrick, Maryland 21701

MARY E. BRUNKOW (187), Division of Molecular and Developmental Biology, Samuel Lunenfeld Research Institute, Mt. Sinai Hospital, Toronto M5G 1X5, Canada

KAREN BUCHKOVICH[1] (119), Cold Spring Harbor Laboratory, Cold Spring Harbor, New York 11724, and Massachusetts General Hospital Cancer Center, Charlestown, Massachusetts 02129

TOM CURRAN (23), Roche Institute of Molecular Biology, Roche Research Center, Nutley, New Jersey 07110

[1]*Present address:* Howard Hughes Medical Institute, Department of Biochemistry, New York University Medical Center, New York, New York 10016

JAMES A. DeCAPRIO (133), The Dana-Farber Cancer Institute, and Harvard Medical School, Boston, Massachusetts 02115

CLAIRE DEES (187), Duke University School of Medicine, Durham, North Carolina 27706

GABI DOEDERLEIN (53), European Molecular Biology Laboratory, D-6900 Heidelberg, Germany

NICHOLAS DYSON (119), Cold Spring Harbor Laboratory, Cold Spring Harbor, New York 11724, and Massachusetts General Hospital Cancer Center, Charlstown, Massachusetts 02129

CATHY A. FINLAY (87), Department of Molecular Biology, Lewis Thomas Laboratory, Princeton University, Princeton, New Jersey 08544-1014

ED HARLOW (119), Cold Spring Harbor Laboratory, Cold Spring Harbor, New York 11724, and Massachusetts General Hospital Cancer Center, Charlestown, Massachusetts 02129

DAVID E. HOUSMAN (147), Center for Cancer Research, Massachusetts Institute of Technology, Cambridge, Massachusetts 02139

QIANJIN HU (119), Cold Spring Harbor Laboratory, Cold Spring Harbor, New York 11724, and Massachusetts General Hospital Cancer Center, Charlestown, Massachusetts 02129

WILLIAM G. KAELIN JR. (133), The Dana-Farber Cancer Institute, and Harvard Medical School, Boston, Massachusetts 02115

FREDERIC J. KAYE (133), National Cancer Institute-Navy Medical Oncology Branch, and Uniformed Services, University of the Health Sciences, Bethesda, Maryland 20814

JACQUELINE LEES (119), Cold Spring Harbor Laboratory, Cold Spring Harbor, New York 11724, and Massachusetts General Hospital Cancer Center, Charlestown, Massachusetts 02129

ARNOLD J. LEVINE (87), Department of Molecular Biology, Lewis Thomas Laboratory, Princeton University, Princeton, New Jersey 08544-1014

DAVID M. LIVINGSTON (133), The Dana-Farber Cancer Institute, and Harvard Medical School, Boston, Massachusetts 02115

PASCALE MACGREGOR (23), Roche Institute of Molecular Biology, Roche Research Center, Nutley, New Jersey 07110

DAVID C. PALLAS (133), The Dana-Farber Cancer Institute, and Harvard Medical School, Boston, Massachusetts 02115

KATHARINE PHILLIPS (187), Thomas Jefferson University School of Medicine, Philadelphia, Pennsylvania 19107

B. FRANKLIN PUGH[2] (201), Howard Hughes Medical Institute, Department of Molecular and Cell Biology, University of California, Berkeley, Berkeley, California 94720

ROBIN S. QUARTIN (87), Department of Molecular Biology, Lewis Thomas Laboratory, Princeton University, Princeton, New Jersey 08544-1014

SHIRLEY M. TILGHMAN (187), Howard Hughes Medical Institute, and Department of Molecular Biology, Princeton University, Princeton, New Jersey 08544

ROBERT TJIAN (201), Howard Hughes Medical Institute, Department of Molecular and Cell Biology, University of California, Berkeley, Berkeley, California 94720

RICHARD TREISMAN (163), Transcription Laboratory, Imperial Cancer Research Fund, Lincoln's Inn Fields, London WC2A 3PX, England

BERT VOGELSTEIN (105), Oncology Center, Johns Hopkins University School of Medicine, Baltimore, Maryland 21231

ROBERT A. WEINBERG (3), Whitehead Institute for Biomedical Research, and Massachusetts Institute of Technology, Department of Biology, Cambridge, Massachusetts 02139

MARTIN ZENKE (53), Institute of Molecular Pathology, A 1030 Vienna, Austria

[2]*Present address:* Department of Molecular and Cell Biology, The Pennsylvania State University, University Park, Pennsylvania 16802

Editor's Foreword

Finding a comprehensive cure for cancer has been a long quest. Individual cancers, at various stages, can be cured by effective therapy in combination with early diagnosis and appropriate staging. Basic science strives to unravel the mysteries of cancer development in a manner that will lead to a broad-based curative attack on the entire process of malignant disease. An area of particular excitement today is understanding the mechanisms by which genes regulate cell division and growth. The Fourteenth Annual Bristol-Myers Squibb Symposium on Cancer Research, entitled "Nuclear Processes and Oncogenes," which took place at the Massachusetts Institute of Technology on September 24–25, 1990, addressed the subject with the help of some of the leading investigators in the world.

This Symposium is part of a major commitment to funding cancer research established by the Bristol-Myers Squibb Company in 1977. In addition to funding these symposia, Bristol-Myers Squibb has provided over $14 million in no-strings-attached grants for cancer research, awarding 29 grants to 26 institutions in the United States and abroad. This represents the largest contribution of unrestricted funds made by a corporation in support of cancer research.

Stephen K. Carter

Foreword

It would have been hard to project, 25 or 30 years ago, that we would one day be able to pinpoint the specific genes responsible for causing different types of cancer. Recent advances in molecular biology and genetics have given us a much greater understanding of how cancers develop and metastasize. And, with scientist's ever-increasing knowledge base will come better tools to treat cancer more effectively.

The work of many of the scientists responsible for these advances is reflected in this volume of papers delivered during the Fourteenth Annual Bristol-Myers Squibb Symposium on Cancer Research, "Nuclear Processes and Oncogenes," held on September 24–25, 1990, at the Massachusetts Institute of Technology. The symposium was organized by Phillip A. Sharp, of Massachusetts Institute of Technology's Center for Cancer Research, in collaboration with Robert A. Weinberg, of the Whitehead Institute for Biomedical Research, and J. Michael Bishop, of the University of California, San Francisco.

In addition to funding Bristol-Myers Squibb cancer symposia since 1977, the company has committed more than $14 million in no-strings-attached grants over those 13 years to support innovative cancer research. This represents the largest contribution of unrestricted funds for cancer research made by any corporation. Twenty-nine of these no-strings-attached grants have been given to 26 institutions in the United States and other countries since the program began.

The centerpiece of the program is the Bristol-Myers Squibb Award for Distinguished Achievement in Cancer Research. The award and a $50,000 prize are presented annually to an individual researcher selected by an independent peer-review committee made up of principal investigators at grant-recipient institutions. The research of three of these distinguished scientists—Ed Harlow, the 1991 award winner; Bert Vogelstein, the 1990 award winner; and Robert Weinberg, the 1984 award winner—is represented in these proceedings.

Since 1977, when the cancer program began, Bristol-Myers Squibb has initiated similar no-strings-attached grant programs in nutrition, orthopedics, neuroscience, pain and, most recently, cardiovascular and infectious disease research. To date, the company has contributed more than $33 million to medical centers and academic research institutions involved in the seven programs.

This fourteenth Bristol-Myers Squibb cancer research symposium volume and those that have preceded it since 1977 are permanent records of the advances in this area that have been made in just thirteen years' time. With each passing year comes new discovery and a vision of the possibilities that lie ahead. Bristol-Myers Squibb is proud to encourage and support that vision through our no-strings-attached research grants program.

Richard L. Gelb

Preface

Cancer is a genetic disease of cells in which the typical tumor cell has suffered five mutational changes. Some mutations activate oncogenes, while others inactivate tumor suppressor genes, and still other mutations may promote the metastatic spread of the malignant cells. As mentioned in Chapter 2 of this volume, some sixty different oncogenes and four tumor suppressor genes have been identified. Only a few of the oncogenes and tumor-suppressor genes occur frequently in common types of human cancers. Among these are the *myc* family of oncogenes and the tumor-suppressor genes retinoblastoma RB and p53. The proteins of all three of these genes are localized to the nucleus and, in the case of *myc,* are almost certainly responsible for the regulation of transcription. It is also possible, and in fact likely, that p53 and retinoblastoma proteins are also transcription factors or interact with proteins that specifically bind DNA. Because the cancer cell differs from a normal cell in alterations of expression of several genes that result in proliferation, migration, and arrests in differentiation, it may be possible to biochemically analyze this disease at the level of regulation of transcription.

The goal of the Fourteenth Annual Bristol-Myers Squibb Symposium on Cancer Research was to codify recent advances in the functions and structures of nuclear proteins encoded by oncogenes and tumor-suppressor genes and to explore the relationship between the biochemical properties of these proteins and regulation of transcription. These two rapidly advancing areas of research, the molecular biology of oncology and mechanisms of regulation of transcription in human cells, could be only partially discussed in a two-day period. Selecting speakers for this task was difficult as there are many excellent scientists in the two fields. The program greatly benefited from the participation of Michael J. Bishop and Robert Weinberg on the organizing committee. I heartily thank these two colleagues for their help.

Cancer will probably not be considered curable within the careers of current scientists and physicians. This task will require the building of a foundation of knowledge, which is well under way, and a transfer of this knowledge and the objective to the next generation who may see the final victory. This symposium on cancer research was held on the campus of Massachusetts Institute of Technology to encourage attendance by students, young physicians, and research fellows. Over 1200 people attended the sessions, most of them young aspiring students and scientists. Many of these young people will take up the challenge of mastering this human disease.

This volume is divided into three parts: nuclear oncogenes, nuclear tumor-suppressor genes, and regulation of transcription. The nuclear oncogenes discussed are primarily *myc, myb, erbA, fos,* and *jun.* Three recently isolated tumor-suppressor genes are reviewed; retinoblastoma (RB), p53, and Wilms. Finally, mechanisms underlying regulation of transcription are discussed in the context of induction of mitogenesis, differentiation, and general transcription.

Phillip A. Sharp

PART I

Nuclear Oncogenes

1

Oncogenes, Tumor-Suppressor Genes, and the Deregulation of Cell Growth: An Overview

ROBERT A. WEINBERG
Whitehead Institute for Biomedical Research
and Massachusetts Institute of Technology
Department of Biology
Cambridge, Massachusetts

I. Introduction

The research field that attempts to describe the molecular biology of cancer is barely 15 years old, yet it has grown so large and diversified that its various component parts are hard to unite in one coherent conceptual scheme. How can the diverse findings about oncogenes and tumor suppressor genes, growth factors, receptors, and second messengers be rationalized? Despite this diversity of topics and research directions, some central principles emerge to provide unifying explanations of the deregulation of growth control seen in cancer cells.

The guiding light here is provided by a focus on intercellular communication and its disruption during cancer pathogenesis. The architecture of a normal tissue is developed and maintained by a complex communication network between its constituent cells. Within this community of cells, cells receive both growth-stimulatory and growth-inhibitory signals from their neighbors. The decisions undertaken by an individual cell concerning growth, differentiation, and quiescence are not made autonomously, but rather depend largely if not totally on cues received from the cell's surroundings as defined by neighboring cells within the tissue. The evolving cancer cell cuts itself loose from such contextual signals and assumes partial or total control over its own growth-regulating decisions. This acquired autonomy is essential to its clonal expansion and can increasingly be explained in molecular and biochemical terms.

One measure of acquired growth autonomy is evidenced by the reduced dependence that cancer cells have on growth-stimulating signals provided by their environment. Tissue culture experiments indicate that normal cells grow only after being stimulated to do so by multiple, distinct growth factors. Various types of cancer cells appear to grow independently of the presence of normally growth factors.

The identity of these growth factors varies from one cell type to another, and the precise number of distinct growth factors normally involved in inducing different cells to divide is still unclear. As an example, certain fibroblasts grown in culture have been shown to require PDGF (platelet-derived growth factor), EGF (epidermal growth factor), and IGF-1 (insulin-like growth factor) before they will emerge from the quiescent G_0 growth state, traverse the G_1 phase of the growth cycle, and initiate DNA synthesis.

Transformed fibroblasts no longer exhibit this extensive dependence on exogenous stimulatory signals. The oncogenes found in many types of tumor cells operate via several different growth-stimulating mechanisms to confer this factor independence. They do so by virtue of the fact that their gene products, the oncoproteins, sit astride the major signaling pathways used by cells to regulate normal cell growth.

From the beginning to the end of mitogen-triggered signaling pathways, oncogene proteins can act potently to deregulate these pathways, causing them to become constitutively activated. In so doing, they obviate the normally required encounters of a growth factor-dependent cell with exogenous mitogens. Cells that carry activated oncogenes are persuaded by these genes that mitogens have been encountered, since these genes and their encoded proteins are able to mimic the signals that a cell experiences when such an encounter indeed takes place.

II. Oncogenes

At least four distinct mechanisms allow oncogene proteins to activate constitutively these signaling pathways. Oncogenes like *sis, hst*-1, and *int*-1 encode growth factors (GFs) that are expressed constitutively and in high amounts. As a consequence, the oncogene-bearing cell releases large amounts of growth factors into its surrounds. Once released, these GFs may then stimulate the growth of the same cell that has just produced them. Such a positive feedback or *autocrine* loop makes encounters with GFs of exogenous origin unnecessary.

The receptors that stud cell surfaces and are used to recognize GFs in the extracellular space may also assume the role of oncoproteins. Having suffered structural alterations or being expressed at higher-than-normal levels, the receptor proteins can flood the cell with mitogenic signals even in the absence of binding ligand. Once again, the presence of exogenous GF has been rendered unnecessary.

These receptors activate complex signaling cascades that begin in the cytoplasm and reach into the nucleus where they converge ultimately on the cell's decision as to whether it should grow, differentiate, or remain quiescent. The proximal signal-transducing proteins that participate in these cascades in the cell cytoplasm may undergo structural change. Having done so, they acquire the ability to emit mitogenic signals, even without prior stimulation by ligand-activated receptors. The *ras, src,* and *abl* oncoproteins are good examples of this.

Finally, in the nucleus we find a number of genes that respond to mitogen stimulation by producing greatly increased amounts of growth-promoting proteins. The *myc, fos,* and *jun* oncogenes represent good examples; their encoded proteins affect growth by regulating banks of responder genes. When undergoing oncogenic activation, these genes acquire an ability to become constitutively expressed, and thus are no longer dependent on mitogen stimulation for increased expression.

III. Tumor-Suppressor Genes

It has been apparent that oncogenes like these provide only part of the answer to the problem of malignant transformation. A rapidly growing corpus of evidence suggests that gene inactivation, rather than deregulation, plays an equally important role in cancer pathogenesis. The genes affected in this way—collectively termed the *tumor suppressor genes*—must act in normal cells to confine or constrain growth. When one of these suffers inactivation, the cell is deprived of a vital component of its braking machinery. As a consequence, its growth continues unabated under conditions where by all rights its proliferation should cease.

This loss disrupts the intercellular signaling network described earlier, but in a fashion quite different from that of oncogenes. As mentioned earlier, cells impose growth inhibition on one another to ensure that no cell within a tissue breaks rank and begins to grow inappropriately. The loss of one or another tumor suppressor gene deprives a cell of its ability to respond appropriately to growth-inhibitory signals, leading in turn to a phenotype similar to that seen in oncogene-transformed cells—runaway growth.

What evidence can be adduced to highlight the importance of this mutual growth inhibition? Most well known is the contact inhibition experienced by nonmalignant cells in tissue culture. Yet another more dramatic case comes from work of Paolo Dotto, who studied the tumorigenicity of *ras* oncogene-transformed mouse skin keratinocytes when implanted on the back of a mouse (Dotto *et al.*, 1988). A pure population of these rapidly expanded into a squamous cell carcinoma. However, when such cells were admixed with untransformed dermal fibroblasts before implantation, only small fibrotic nodules ensued. These dermal fibroblasts exist in close contact with keratinocytes in the intact mouse skin, and their presence clearly suppresses the growth ability of the oncogene-transformed keratinocytes. Accordingly, it appears that tumor cells like this one need to acquire the strong growth impetus provided by an oncogene like *ras*, and at the same time must escape environmental growth inhibition provided by neighboring cells in order to form tumors.

Escape from such inhibition resulted from the artifice of physically segregating these cells from the source of the inhibition, the dermal fibroblasts. A less artificial means to achieve this loss could come from a breakdown of the cell's signal-transducing machinery that confers responsiveness to such inhibition. One clue to the nature of this signalling machinery comes from work on the retinoblastoma (*Rb*) gene whose homozygous inactivation triggers the rare eye tumor of childhood. The tumor can arise by two routes, both resulting in the inactivation of the two chromosome 13-associated *Rb* gene copies. In familial cases, a child acquires a defective *Rb* allele from one or another parent; accordingly, all cells in the retina are effectively hemizygous for Rb. The second allele can then be lost in a retinal cell through somatic mutation. In sporadic cases of retinoblastoma, both gene copies are lost through somatic mutation (Knudson, 1971). This required loss of both copies clearly indicates that either intact Rb gene copy suffices to program normal growth, and that this gene acts in one or another way to constrain proliferation.

The *Rb* protein is phosphorylated and is found in the nucleus, suggesting a role in regulation of gene expression, but its precise function is not yet well established. One clue to its mechanism of action has come from study of DNA tumor viruses, initially adenovirus type 5. Its E1A oncogene is able to induce a number of distinct changes in cell phenotype, including immortalization, and is able to collaborate with a *ras* oncogene in cell transformation. Two groups have found that the E1A oncoproteins are able to complex with at least six different host cell proteins, ostensibly altering the function of each and in this way achieving cell transformation (Yee and Branton, 1985; Harlow *et al.*, 1986). As Harlow's group has found, one of the host cell targets of E1A is the transformed cell's *Rb* protein (Whyte *et al.*, 1988). Moreover, mutations in the E1A protein that compromise its ability to complex with $p105^{Rb}$ also knock out its transforming powers (Whyte *et al.*, 1989).

IV. Interactions of Oncogenes and Tumor-Suppressor Gene Activities

How does this fit in with the above-described role of $p105^{Rb}$ as a transducer of inhibitory signals? Harold Moses' laboratory has shown that the much-studied growth-inhibitory factor TGF-β is potent in its ability to shut down transcription of the *myc* gene in keratinocytes with an associated cessation of growth. But in cells that carry the E1A or SV40 viral oncoproteins, this shutdown is not achieved by TGF-β, ostensibly because the oncoproteins sequester the

Rb protein, thereby interdicting this signaling pathway (Pietenpol *et al.*, 1990). Significantly, mutants of the viral proteins that fail to bind $p105^{Rb}$ also fail to interdict the TGF-β-mediated suppression of *myc* expression. All this is consistent with a model in which $p105^{Rb}$ acts as a critical link in the signaling pathway that is responsible for shutting down genes like *myc*.

If the model that Rb acts to repress nuclear protooncogenes is extended and fleshed out in biochemical detail, this will provide a new means of understanding multistep carcinogenesis and oncogene collaboration. As is now well documented, cellular oncogenes like *myc* and *ras* are able to collaborate to transform primary into tumorigenic cells. The biological basis of this has been difficult to rationalize. These results, still preliminary, provide a means to conceptualize this.

As argued earlier, oncogenes like *ras* supply gratuitous mitogenic signals to cells, thereby relieving their dependence on exogenous growth factors. But how do *myc* and its analogs function? *Ras* oncogene-transformed cells are unable to expand clonally in the presence of formal neighbors; the presence of a *myc* oncogene enables them to do so. This suggests that the constitutively expressed *myc* gene (i.e., oncogenic form) is able to drive cell growth under conditions in which the normal *myc* protooncogene would be shut down in response to physiologic growth-inhibitory signals received by the cell. The *myc* oncogene would therefore seem to enable the cell to ignore and override environmental inhibitory signals.

But *myc* oncogenes are only rarely seen in tumor cells. Thus, the physiologic state achieved by *myc* oncogene activation must be mimicked by other changes in the cell. The most attractive means of doing so is to deregulate *myc* expression through a disruption of its *trans*-acting upstream transcriptional regulators. In many tumors, constitutive *myc* expression, uncoupled from physiologic signals, may well be achieved through deletion of proteins like $p105^{Rb}$. In virus-transformed cells, the same result can occur through inactivation of $p105^{Rb}$ at the hands of oncoproteins like E1A, SV40 large T, and the human papillomavirus E7 protein, all of which bind and apparently sequester $p105^{Rb}$ (DeCaprio *et al.*, 1988; Dyson *et al.*, 1989). This may explain how the viral oncoproteins are able to act as analogs of *myc* in oncogene-collaboration tests. By deregulating *myc*, they create the same affect as *cis*-acting mutations in the *myc* gene itself.

All this would seem to hint at a larger theme in tumor biology: that cell transformation depends both on gratuitous mitogenic signals and the loss of responsiveness to environmental growth-inhibitory signals. The complex process of multistep tumorigenesis may eventually be understood in terms of a small number of central, basic principles. Prominent among them will be the activation of oncogenes and the inactivation of tumor suppressor genes.

References

DeCaprio, J. A., Ludlow, J. W., Figge, J., Shew, J-Y., Huang, C-M., Lee, W-H., Marsilio, E., Paucha, E., and Livingston, D. M. (1988). SV40 Large tumor antigen forms a specific complex with the product of the retinoblastoma susceptibility gene. *Cell* **54,** 275–283.

Dotto, G. P., Weinberg, R. A., and Ariza, A. (1988). Malignant transformation of mouse primary keratinocytes by Harvey sarcoma virus and its modulation by surrounding normal cells. *Proc. Natl. Acad. Sci. U.S.A.* **85,** 6389–6393.

Dyson, N., Howley, P. M., Münger, K., and Harlow, E. (1989). The human papilloma virus-16 E7 oncoprotein is able to bind to the retinoblastoma gene product. *Science* **243,** 934–937.

Harlow, E., Whyte, P., Franza, B. R., Jr., and Schley, C. (1986). Association of adenovirus early-region 1A proteins with cellular polypeptides. *Mol. Cell. Biol.,* **6,** 1579–1589.

Knudson, A. G., Jr. (1971). Mutation and cancer: Statistical study of retinoblastoma. *Proc. Natl. Acad. Sci. U.S.A.* **68,** 820–823.

Pietenpol, J. A., Stein, R. W., Moran, E., Yaciuk, P., Schlegel, R., Lyons, R. M., Pittelkow, M. R., Münger, K., Howley, P. M., and Moses, H. L. (1990). TGF-β1 inhibition of c-*myc* transcription and growth in keratinocytes is abrogated by viral transforming proteins with pRB-binding domains. *Cell* **61,** 777–785.

Whyte, P., Buchkovich, K. J., Horowitz, J. M., Friend, S. H., Raybuck, J., Weinberg, R. A., and Harlow, E. (1988). Association between an oncogene and an anti-oncogene: The adenovirus E1A proteins bind to the retinoblastoma gene product. *Nature (London)* **334,** 124–129.

Whyte, P., Williamson, N. M., and Harlow, E. (1989). Cellular targets for transformation by the adenovirus E1A proteins. *Cell* **56,** 67–75.

Yee, S., and Branton, P. (1985). Detection of cellular proteins associated with human adenovirus type 5 early region 1A polypeptide. *Virology* **147,** 142–153.

2

The Functions of *MYB* and *MYC*

J. MICHAEL BISHOP

Departments of Microbiology and Immunology and Biochemistry and Biophysics; and The G. W. Hooper Research Foundation University of California, San Francisco San Francisco, California

I. Introduction

Two sorts of genetic damage lie at the heart of tumorigenesis: dominant, with targets known colloquially as protooncogenes; and recessive, with targets known variously as tumor-suppressor genes, growth-suppressor genes, recessive oncogenes, or antioncogenes (Bishop, 1987). Protooncogenes were first uncovered by studying the

NUCLEAR PROCESSES
AND ONCOGENES

TABLE I

Protooncogenes with Nuclear Products

Protooncogene	Function[a]
ERBA	Transcription factor (thyroid hormone receptor)
EVI-1	Transcription factor (?)
ETS-1	Transcription factor
ETS-2	Transcription factor
FOS	Transcription factor (AP-1)
JUN	Transcription factor (AP-1)
MYB	Transcription factor
MYC	Transcription factor (?)
NMYC	Transcription factor (?)
REL	Transcription factor (resembles NFKB)
SKI	?
SPI-1	Transcription factor (PU.1)

[a]Assignment of function is based on experimental test and/or structural resemblance to previously identified factors.

cellular origins of retroviral oncogenes, but the roster has since been expanded by diverse lines of enquiry (Varmus, 1989). The tally has now reached sixty or more, although some of the loci have been authenticated by weak inference only (for a recent compilation, see Varmus, 1989); the definition of protooncogene has become more expansive, subsuming any gene with the potential for conversion to an oncogene, by either natural or experimental means.

A still-growing number of protooncogenes encode nuclear proteins (Table I). Study of these genes has provided access to the nuclear apparatus that orchestrates the genetic response during cellular proliferation and differentiation. Five of these genes represent previously recognized transcription factors or close kin; at least six others may encode transcription factors encountered only through the study of protooncogenes (see Table I). Modulation of gene expression is frequently an important ramification of intracellular signaling and plays a vital role in the control of cellular proliferation (Rollins and Stiles, 1989). It comes as no surprise, then, that the malfunction of at least some transcription factors can elicit neoplastic growth.

TABLE II

The *MYB* Gene Family

	Locus		
Organism	*MYB*	*A-MYB*	*B-MYB*
Drosophila	+	−	−
Chicken	+	+	+
Mouse	+	+	+
Human	+	+	+

II. The Protooncogenes *MYB* and *MYC*

The protooncogenes *MYB* and *MYC* were encountered first as oncogenes in retroviruses (for a recent review of these genes and their products, see Cole, 1990). Both are prototypes for small gene families whose sizes are not yet certain, and most of whose members remain unstudied (Tables II and III). We have no insight into the selective pressures that gave rise to this diversification. The oncogenes derived from *MYB* and *MYC* have distinctive tumorigenicities, although both can cause leukemias in the myeloid lineage. Both genes encode nuclear phosphoproteins with short half-lives, properties that bespeak possible roles in the regulation of cellular function. The product of *MYB* binds to a degenerate but specific site in DNA (Oehler *et al.*, 1990), whereas the claims for specific binding of *MYC* protein to DNA remain less secure (Ariga *et al.*, 1989). Recent work has brought the products of both *MYB* and *MYC* into better focus. These proteins can regulate transcription in one way or another, and they appear to be involved in the proliferation of vertebrate cells.

TABLE III

The MYC Gene Family

CMYC
NMYC
LMYC
LMYC (pseudogene)
RMYC
PMYC
BMYC

TABLE IV

Formation of Homo-Oligomers by MYC Protein

Motifs in MYC allele	Dimers	Tetramers
Helix–loop–helix and zipper	+	+
Helix–loop–helix only	+	–
Zipper only	+	–

III. The Structure of *MYC* Protein

MYC encodes two closely related nuclear proteins (Hann *et al.*, 1988). The biochemical function of these proteins remains uncertain, although roles in both transcription (Kaddurah-Daouk *et al.*, 1987) and DNA replication (Ariga *et al.*, 1989) have been suggested. In particular, the carboxyterminal domains of the proteins contain three structural motifs that suggest a role in transcription: a domain rich in basic amino acids, a helix–loop–helix configuration, and a leucine zipper. Mutations in each of these regions are especially likely to inactivate the biological function of *MYC*, although the amino-terminal half of the molecule also contains regions essential for activity (Stone *et al.*, 1987).

The leucine zipper and helix–loop–helix motif have been implicated in the genesis of multimeric proteins, and the formation of these oligomers is typically essential for function (Johnson and McKnight, 1989). Accordingly, the products of *MYC* form dimers and tetramers when synthesized *in vitro* and allowed to interact (Dang *et al.*, 1989, and unpublished data of G. Ramsay and J. M. B.). Deletion of either the leucine zipper or the helix–loop–helix eliminated the formation of tetramers, but had no effect on the formation of dimers (Table IV). It appears that either of the interactive domains can mediate dimerization, but that tetramers form only if both domains are available for use. These findings were made *in vitro* and may conceal a more complex reality *in vivo*. It seems possible that within the cell, one of the interactive domains is used to form homodimers, whereas the other is used to form an additional complex with a heterologous protein or proteins, required for function and perhaps responsible for specificity.

IV. The Effect of *MYC* on Transcription

In order to explore the function of *MYC*, we have created alleles of the gene whose products are regulated by one or another steroid hormone (Eilers *et al.*, 1989). For example, a chimera composed of the hormone-binding domain of the human estrogen receptor fused to the carboxy-terminus of the *MYC* protein displayed complete dependence on estrogen in the transformation of established rat fibroblasts. Since these cells are devoid of the normal estrogen receptor, all effects of the hormone can be attributed to the action of the conditional *MYC* protein.

We have used an estrogen-inducible version of *MYC* to identify a cellular gene whose transcription can be greatly augmented by the action of *MYC* (Eilers *et al.*, 1990). Induction of transcription by *MYC* was maximal within several hours, was effected by changing the rate of initiation, and did not require intervening protein synthesis. From these findings, we concluded that the product of *MYC* can act directly on the transcriptional apparatus, in accord with inferences based on the structure of the protein. But we know nothing of the details by which that action occurs.

The gene whose control by *MYC* we uncovered encodes the protein known as α-prothymosin (Eilers *et al.*, 1990). Prothymosin was at first believed to be a precursor to a thymic growth factor. In the interim, views have changed (as summarized in Eilers *et al.*, 1990). First, the effect of thymosin and prothymosin on T cells may be nonspecific. Second, the structure of prothymosin carries no hallmark of a secretory protein. Instead, the protein has been found in the nucleus and contains a functioning nuclear localization signal. Third, prothymosin displays structural kinship with a variety of acidic nuclear proteins, including high mobility group proteins, nucleolin, a cofactor for RNA polymerase I, and proliferating cell nuclear antigen (PCNA), an auxiliary factor for DNA polymerase δ. None of these proteins has an assigned function, but it is suspected that their acidic domains may help to modulate chromatin structure for sundry purposes. Fourth, expression of prothymosin is apparently restricted to proliferating cells and is induced by the application of serum to quiescent cells—as anticipated for a gene under the control of *MYC*. These findings combine to suggest that prothymosin itself may play a role in the vertebrate cell cycle, a suggestion that acquires further credence from our finding that transcription of the prothymosin gene is under the control of *MYC*. Whatever the function of its product, the prothymosin gene can be used to explore the mechanism by which *MYC* influences transcription.

V. The *MYB* Protein as a Transcription Factor

The product of *MYB* can activate transcription in diverse settings (Cole, 1990). Two regions of the *MYB* protein have been implicated in the activation: a repeated domain near the amino-terminus that is responsible for DNA binding; and a sequence of 35 to 50 amino acids within the heart of the protein that is essential and sufficient for transcriptional activation when tethered to the DNA-binding domain. The activation sequence is moderately acidic but otherwise undistinctive, bearing no explicit resemblance to other known activators of transcription (Johnson and McKnight, 1989).

Recent work has identified one cellular gene that appears to be under the control of *MYB* in a natural setting (Ness *et al.*, 1989). In an effort to find additional such genes, we have created an estrogen-inducible allele of *MYB*, similar to that described above for *MYC* (unpublished work of Sabine Schirm and the author). The hormone-binding domain from the estrogen receptor was fused to the amino-terminus of the *MYB* protein. The chimeric protein is biochemically inactive in the absence of estrogen, but regains full transcriptional activation in the presence of hormone. These findings demonstrate that the hormone-binding domain exerts direct control over the biochemical action of the *MYB* protein and expands the variety of proteins that have been placed under the control of a steroid hormone (for previous examples, see Eilers *et al.*, 1989). The conditional allele of *MYB* represents a device with which to seek genes under the control of *MYB*.

VI. *MYB* and *MYC* in the Cell Cycle

The return of resting cells from G_0 to the active cell-division cycle is accompanied by manifold changes in gene expression (Rollins and Stiles, 1989). The earliest changes occur within the first few hours and involve a large battery of *early-response* or *immediate-early* genes, among which are the protooncogenes *FOS* and *MYC* (Fig. 1). Expression of *MYB* is activated at a later time, reaching a maximum

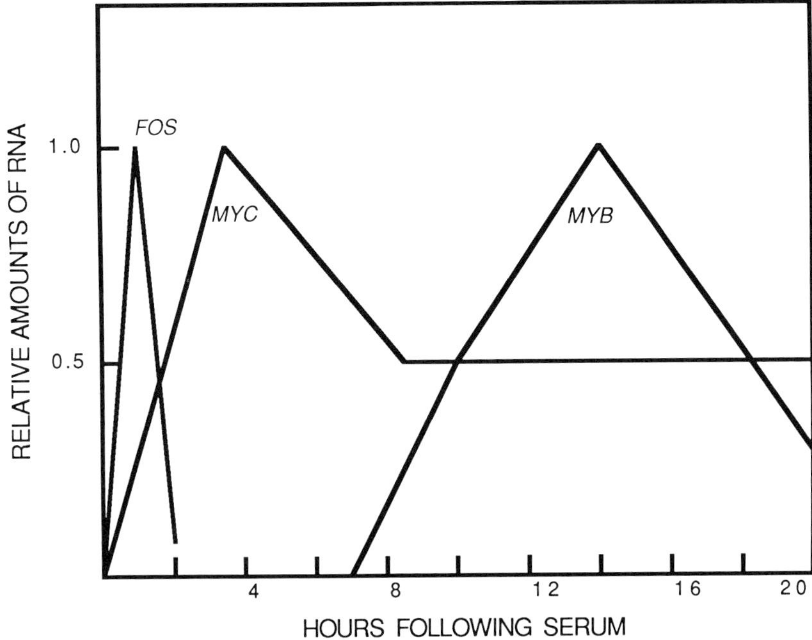

Fig. 1. Activation of protooncogenes during the cellular response to serum. The diagram is a stylized portrayal of fluctuations in the levels of RNA following stimulation of quiescent rat fibroblasts with serum. The portrayal is in relative terms. The absolute responses vary greatly. For example, the response of *MYC* is ca. 400-fold greater than that of *MYB*.

shortly before the onset of the S phase. At first glance, activation of the early-response genes seems to take the form of a temporal sequence or cascade. In reality, however, none of these genes is likely to be under the control of another, since they all are induced by serum in the absence of protein synthesis (summarized in Rollins and Stiles, 1989).

We have used an estrogen-inducible allele of *MYC* to explore the role of *MYC* in cellular proliferation. Quiescent cells carrying the inducible version of *MYC* protein could be returned to the cell cycle by stimulation with estrogen (Fig. 2). The cells proceeded through M, and even initiated a second round of division, despite the absence of any exogenous growth factors (Eilers *et al.*, 1990). The reentry into the cell cycle occurred without the induction of *FOS* (Fig. 2) or other immediate-early genes. The S phase induced by estrogen began ca. 3 hr earlier than that induced by serum, a period that corresponds

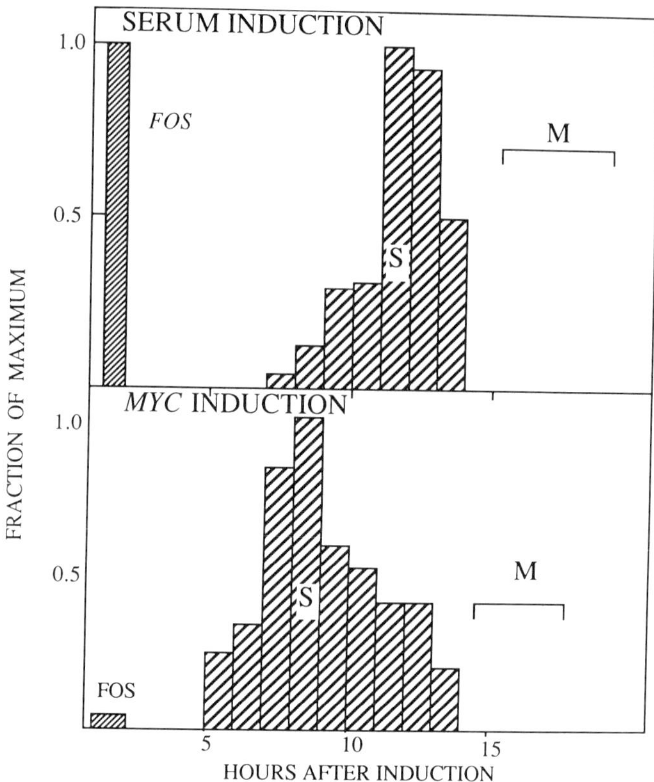

Fig. 2. Induction of the cell-division cycle by serum and *MYC*. Quiescent RAT-1A fibroblasts were stimulated to divide with either serum or an ectopic allele of *MYC* whose product was under the control of estrogen (see Eilers *et al.*, 1989, 1990). The diagram illustrates the relative amounts of *FOS* RNA present in cells 30 min following stimulation, the occurrence of S phase (as measured by incorporation of labeled thymidine), and the occurrence of mitosis (detected by flow cytometry).

approximately to the time required for induction of *MYC* itself by serum (Fig. 2). These findings suggest that the action of *MYC* can be sufficient to elicit the complete cell cycle, bypassing the need for earlier events in the recovery from quiescence.

The transcriptional response to *MYC* has not been explored in detail, but among the events that follow activation of *MYC* are the induction of prothymosin, PCNA, and *MYB*. These inductions occur in resting cells stimulated by either serum or the estrogen-regulated allele of *MYC*. The induction of prothymosin is a direct event (see above and Eilers *et al.*, 1990), whereas the inductions of PCNA and

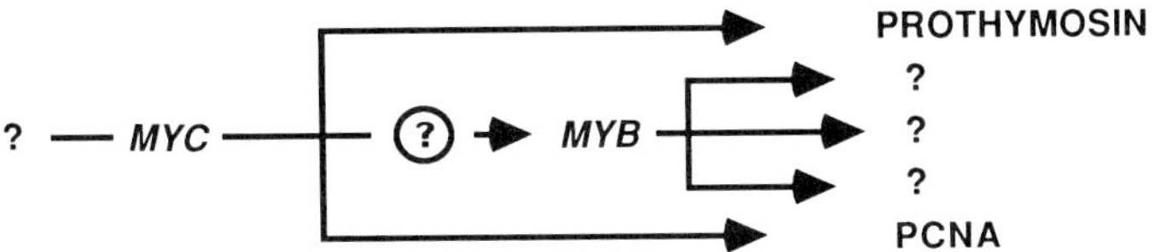

Fig. 3. Transcriptional response to growth factors: a spreading signal. The diagram illustrates how the immediate response to *MYC* and the eventual induction of *MYB* can diversify the transcriptional response to serum growth factors. The mechanism by which the expression of *MYC* is induced is not known, nor is the nature of the connection between *MYC* and MYB.

MYB have yet to be appropriately characterized. Prothymosin and PCNA represent acidic proteins that may contribute to the modulation of chromatin structure. In contrast, the *MYB* protein is apparently a transcription factor whose induction by *MYC* raises a provocative image: the control of *MYB* by *MYC*, whether direct or indirect, exemplifies how the activation of one transcription factor can create a signal that will eventually spread to encompass many genes (Fig. 3). A spreading signal of this sort provides a potential explanation of how the action of a single gene (in this event, *MYC*) can trigger the cell-division cycle.

VII. The Function of *MYB* in *Drosophila melanogaster*

Much of what we know about the function of protooncogenes has been learned from the study of homogeneous populations of cells in culture rather than of tissues in organisms. The fruit fly, *Drosophila melanogaster*, provides an opportunity to remedy this deficiency through genetic analysis. A wide variety of protooncogenes are represented in *D. melanogaster* (Hoffmann, 1989), including a reasonable facsimile of *MYB* (but regrettably, not of *MYC*) (Katzen *et al.*, 1985). The expression of *MYB* occurs throughout the development of the fruit fly, principally (but not exclusively) in proliferating tissues (unpublished results of A. Katzen and J. M. B.)—in accord with the inference that *MYB* may be involved in the cell-division cycle. That inference has been reinforced by the first results from genetic analysis.

A mutant allele of drosophila *MYB* has been identified and partially characterized (Table V). The allele is recessive, hypomorphic (i.e., not completely inactive), and partially penetrant in a tem-

TABLE V

Pleiotropism of a Recessive Mutation in *Drosophila myb*

Hypomorphic (not null) allele: partial temperature dependence
Maternal effects on embryogenesis and oogenesis
Lethal effects in embryos, larvae, and pupae
Diverse abnormalities in development, including abdominal cuticle and wings
Impaired flight: ? neuromuscular defect
Diminished female (and male?) fertility
An underlying defect (?): diminished cell division in imaginal lineages

perature-dependent manner. Homozygosity for the mutation confers diverse phenotypic effects on the organism, originating as both maternal and zygotic influences. Prominent among these are defects in oogenesis, embryogenesis, and later development, many of which are lethal when fully expressed.

The underlying defect may be a diminution of cell division in various embryological lineages. The first clue to this defect came from the observation that the wings of homozygous mutant adults, raised at the relatively permissive temperature of 18°, have one half the number of wing bristles and, presumably, one half the number of cells found in the wings of wild-type flies. Flight of mutant adults is also impaired, probably by a neuromuscular defect. The availability of this mutant will facilitate isolation of more mutations in drosophila *MYB* and the use of genetic analysis to dissect the signaling pathways into which *MYB* is integrated.

VIII. Conclusion

The potential of protooncogenes to participate in tumorigenesis arises from the fact that their protein products are relays in the elaborate biochemical circuitry that governs the phenotype of vertebrate cells (Bishop, 1987): polypeptide hormones that act on the surface of the cell, receptors for these hormones, proteins that convey signals from the receptors to the deeper recesses of the cell, and nuclear functions that orchestrate the genetic response to afferent commands. Diverse lines of enquiry have brought these relays into view, but the study of protooncogenes has been among the richest sources. That tenet is illustrated well by *MYB* and *MYC*. Both genes apparently encode transcription factors that have not been encountered in any other venue. Both have been implicated in the proliferation of vertebrate cells, and *MYC* in particular seems to be a nexus for the signaling that arouses quiescent cells in response to growth factors.

Recent times have produced invigorating insights into the division cycle of the eukaryotic cell. The insights have illuminated two elements of that cycle: the signaling pathways that elicit and suppress the cycle (Rollins and Stiles, 1989); and the biochemical oscillator that drives the cycle (Norbury and Nurse, 1989). For the moment, we do not know how these two elements intersect. Pursuit of *MYB* and *MYC* may help solve the puzzle.

Acknowledgments

I thank my several colleagues named in the text for permission to cite unpublished data and for help with the illustrations. Lynn Vogel provided valuable assistance with the manuscript. Work in my laboratory is supported by Grant No. CA 44338 from the National Institutes of Health and by funds from the G. W. Hooper Research Foundation.

References

Ariga, H., Imamura, Y., and Iguchiariga, S. M. M. (1989). DNA replication origin and transcriptional enhancer in c-*myc* gene share the c-*myc* protein binding sequences. *EMBO J.* **8**, 4273–4279.

Bishop, J. M. (1987). The molecular genetics of cancer. *Science* **235**, 305–311.

Cole, M. D. (1990). The *myb* and *myc* nuclear oncogenes as transcriptional activators. *Curr. Opin. Cell Biol.* **2**, 502–508.

Dang, C. V., McGuire, M., Buckmire, M., and Lee, W. M. F. (1989). Involvement of the "leucine zipper" region in the oligomerization and transforming activity of human c-*myc* protein. *Nature (London)* **337**, 664–666.

Eilers, M., Picard, D., Yamamoto, K. R., and Bishop, J. M. (1989). Chimaeras of *myc* oncoprotein and steroid receptors cause hormone-dependent transformation of cells. *Nature (London)* **340**, 66–68.

Eilers, M., Schirm, S., and Bishop, J. M. (1990). The MYC protein activates transcription of the α-prothymosin gene. Manuscript submitted.

Hann, S. R., King, M. W., Bentley, D. L., Anderson, C. W., and Eisenman, R. N. (1988). A non-AUG translational initiation in c-*myc* exon 1 generates an N-terminally distinct protein whose synthesis is disrupted in Burkitt's lymphomas. *Cell* **52**, 185–195.

Hoffman, F. M. (1989). Roles of *Drosophila* protooncogene and growth factor homologs during development of the fly. *Curr. Top. Microbiol. Immunol.* **147,** 1–29.

Johnson, P. F., and McKnight, S. L. (1989). Eukaryotic transcriptional regulatory proteins. *Annu. Rev. Biochem.* **58,** 799–841.

Kaddurah-Daouk, R., Greene, J. M., Baldwin, A. S., Jr., and Kingston, R. E. (1987). Activation and repression of mammalian gene expression by the c-*myc* protein. *Genes Devel.* **1,** 347–358.

Katzen, A. L., Kornberg, T. B., and Bishop, J. M. (1985). Isolation of the protooncogene c-*myb* from *D. melanogaster. Cell* **41,** 449–456.

Ness, S. A., Marknell, A., and Graf, T. (1989). The v-*myb* oncogene product binds to and activates the promyelocyte-specific MIM-1 gene. *Cell* **59,** 1115–1125.

Norbury, C. J., and Nurse, P. (1989). Control of the higher eukaryote cell cycle by p34^{cdc2} homologues. *Biochim. Biophys. Acta.* **989,** 85–95.

Oehler, T., Arnold, H., Biedenkapp, H., and Klempnauer, K.-H. (1990). Characterization of the v-*myb* DNA binding domain. *Nucleic Acids Res.* **18,** 173–1710.

Rollins, B. J., and Stiles, C. D. (1989). Serum-inducible genes. *Adv. Cancer Res.* **53,** 1–32.

Stone, J., de Lange, T., Ramsay, G., Jakobovits, E., Bishop, J. M., Varmus, H., and Lee, W. (1987). Definition of regions in human c-*myc* that are involved in transformation and nuclear localization. *Mol. Cell. Biol.* **7,** 1697–1709.

Varmus, H. (1989). An historical overview of oncogenes. *In* "Oncogenes and the Molecular Origins of Cancer" (R. A. Weinberg, ed.), pp. 3–44. Cold Spring Harbor Laboratory Press, New York.

3

Transcriptional Regulation by Fos and Jun

TOM CURRAN, CORY ABATE, AND PASCALE MACGREGOR

Roche Institute of Molecular Biology
Roche Research Center
Nutley, New Jersey

I. Introduction

Long-term cellular responses to environmental cues are controlled by a complex network of intracellular signaling processes. Over the past several years, it has become clear that protooncogenes, the cellular homologs of retroviral oncogenes, operate at focal points of these signal-transduction pathways. Their protein products include growth factors, cell-surface receptors, protein kinases, and G proteins (for reviews see Reddy *et al.*, 1988). In addition, a subset of protooncogenes function as nuclear third messengers that regulate gene expression in response to cell-surface stimulation. Among these are c-*fos* and c-*jun*, protooncogenes that are induced by a great variety of signaling events. Their products, Fos and Jun, function cooperatively to regulate the expression of target genes that contain activator protein (AP-1) DNA-binding sites (Curran and Franza, 1988). Here we describe some of our recent studies that concern the dimerization, DNA binding, and transcriptional properties of Fos and Jun using highly purified polypeptides.

II. The Fos–Jun–AP-1 Connection

The intimate association between Fos, Jun, and the AP-1 binding site was uncovered as a result of several independent lines of research (reviewed in Curran and Franza, 1988). c-*fos*, the cellular homolog of the transforming gene carried by the FBJ and FBR murine sarcoma viruses (Curran and Teich, 1982a; Curran *et al.*, 1983; Curran and Verma, 1984), encodes a nuclear phosphoprotein that forms a stable complex with another nuclear protein originally termed p39 (Curran and Teich, 1982b; Curran *et al.*, 1984, 1985). p39 has now been identified as the product of the protooncogene c-*jun* (Rauscher *et al.*, 1988a). Whereas c-*fos* is expressed at low basal levels in most cell types, its expression is rapidly and transiently induced by a variety of agents associated with mitogenesis, differentiation, and neuronal stimulation (Fig. 1) (reviewed in Curran, 1988). These features, along with the observations that Fos is associated with chromatin (Sambucetti and Curran, 1986; Renz *et al.*, 1987), and that v-*fos* exhibits a transcriptional transactivation property (Setoyama *et al.*, 1986), led to the hypothesis that Fos functions in coupling extracellular stimuli to long-term cellular responses by regulating gene expression (Curran and Morgan, 1987).

The first definitive link between oncogenes and transcription factors was the report of a sequence similarity between v-*jun* and the DNA-binding domain of the yeast transcriptional regulator, GCN4

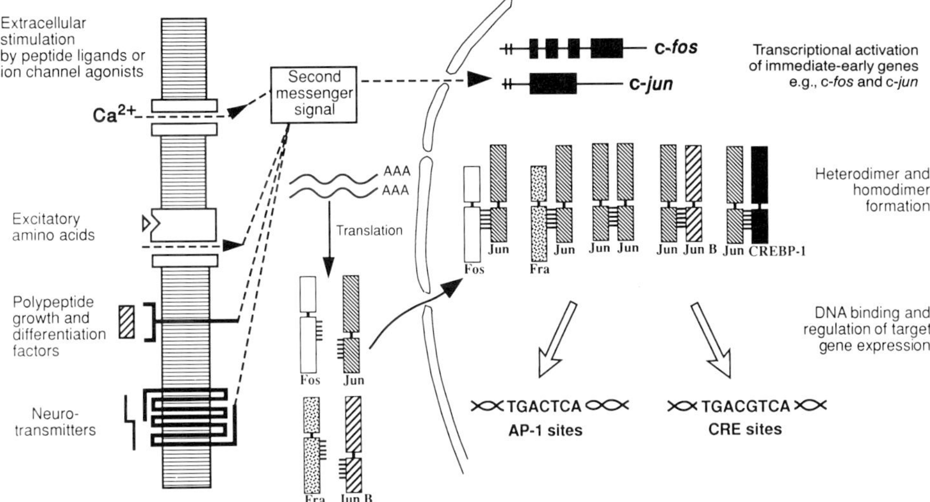

Fig. 1. Signal transduction in the nucleus. c-*fos* and c-*jun* are induced in response to a variety of extracellular signals. Their protein products, Fos and Jun, and the products of *fos*-related genes (Fra) and *jun*-related genes (JunB) form homodimeric complexes in the nucleus that interact with AP-1 sites and CRE sites. Jun can also form heterodimeric complexes with a cyclic AMP-responsive element binding protein, CRE-BP1 that interacts with the CRE site. Reprinted with permission from Curran *et al.,* 1990).

(Vogt *et al.,* 1987). Indeed, the homologous region of Jun was found to be functionally interchangeable with the DNA-binding region of the yeast factor (Struhl, 1987). The recognition site for GCN4 is closely related to the mammalian regulatory element known as the AP-1 binding site (Hill *et al.,* 1986; Hope and Struhl, 1987; Lee *et al.,* 1987a,b). This site has also been identified in phorbol ester-responsive genes and is often referred to as a TPA-responsive site (TRE) (Angel *et al.,* 1987; Lee *et al.,* 1987b). Initial studies identified Jun in preparations of AP-1 binding activity and demonstrated that Jun could interact with the AP-1 binding site (Bohman *et al.,* 1987; Bos *et al.,* 1988). This led to the designation of Jun as *the* AP-1 binding protein. However, it soon became apparent that this early definition was too narrow. The AP-1 site is present in numerous genes that are responsive to a variety of agents in addition to phorbol esters (Curran and Franza, 1988). Moreover, AP-1 binding activity comprises a complex mixture of proteins in addition to Jun, including several Jun- and Fos-related proteins (Franza *et al.,* 1988; Rauscher *et al.,* 1988a).

The first hint of an association of Fos with the AP-1 binding site came from the observation that Fos antisera inhibited the DNA-binding activity associated with a regulatory element from the adipocyte gene, ap-2 (Distel *et al.*, 1987). Subsequently, the critical DNA sequence in this element that interacted with Fos was shown to be the AP-1 binding site (Rauscher *et al.*, 1988b). It is now clear that AP-1 DNA-binding activity contains Fos and Jun as well as several related and unrelated proteins (Franza *et al.*, 1988; Bohmann *et al.*, 1988; Curran *et al.*, 1988). The identification of Jun as the Fos-binding protein, p39 (Rauscher *et al.*, 1988a) prompted the suggestion that Fos and Jun interact as a heterodimeric complex with the AP-1 binding site (Fig. 1). This hypothesis was confirmed using Fos and Jun proteins translated *in vitro* in rabbit reticulocyte lysates (Rauscher *et al.*, 1988c; Nakabeppu *et al.*, 1988; Halazonetis *et al.*, 1988). Furthermore, these studies established that Fos and Jun interact cooperatively with the AP-1 site in the form of a heterodimer. Jun, but not Fos, can interact with the AP-1 site on its own in the form of a homodimeric complex. However, the Fos–Jun complex interacts with a higher apparent affinity owing to an enhanced stability of the heterodimeric complex with DNA (Rauscher *et al.*, 1988c). Fos and Jun also interact with a related DNA site termed the cyclic AMP (cAMP)-responsive element (CRE) (Rauscher *et al.*, 1988c). Several genes related to *fos* and *jun* have now been identified (Cohen and Curran, 1988; Hirai *et al.*, 1989; Ryder *et al.*, 1988; Zerial *et al.*, 1989; Nishina *et al.*, 1990; Matsui *et al.*, 1990), and their protein products form heterodimeric complexes that have DNA-binding properties similar to those of the Fos–Jun complex (Cohen *et al.*, 1989; Nakabeppu *et al.*, 1988; Zerial *et al.*, 1989). The cooperative nature of the Fos–Jun complex is also reflected in a synergistic stimulation of transcription measured in transient transfection assays using reporter genes containing AP-1 binding sites (Lucibello *et al.*, 1988; Sassone-Corsi *et al.*, 1988; Chui *et al.*, 1988; Sonnenberg *et al.*, 1989).

The domains of Fos and Jun that are required for DNA binding and dimerization have been defined by mutagenesis studies using proteins translated in reticulocyte lysates (Kouzarides and Ziff, 1988; Gentz *et al.*, 1989; Turner and Tjian, 1989). This region, contained within the leucine-zipper domain and an adjacent basic region (Fig. 1), is highly conserved among the *fos* and *jun* gene families (Abate and Curran, 1990). The leucine zipper consists of a heptad repeat of leucines that lie along one face of an α-helix and form a dimerization interface. Fos and Jun dimerize via a parallel configuration of these helical regions (Gentz *et al.*, 1989; O'Shea *et al.*, 1989) in a structure that is similar to a coiled-coil. Dimerization brings into appropriate juxtaposition basic regions adjacent to the zipper in both Fos and Jun that contact DNA (Gentz *et al.*, 1989; Kouzarides and Ziff, 1988; Turner and Tjian, 1989; Abate *et al.*, 1990a). The leucine-zipper domain is sufficient for appropriate heterodimer formation as indicated by domain swap studies (Kouzarides and Ziff, 1989; Seller and Struhl, 1989; Nakabeppu and Nathans, 1989; Neuberg *et al.*, 1989; Cohen and Curran, 1990). In addition to conservation of leucine residues, the zipper region contains other amino acids that are highly conserved among either the Fos or Jun families (Abate and Curran, 1990). These amino acids most likely contribute to the preferential heterodimeric association of Fos and Jun. Although the zipper is the primary dimerization domain, and the basic region is the primary DNA-binding domain, amino acids outside of these regions contribute to both dimerization and DNA binding (Cohen and Curran, 1990).

III. Expression and Purification of Fos and Jun in *Escherichia coli*

The studies reviewed established that Fos and Jun function in transcriptional regulation and defined the structural features of these proteins that contribute to dimerization and DNA binding. However, a precise biochemical characterization using impure protein preparations obtained by *in vitro* translation or by oligonucleotide affinity chromatography is not feasible. Therefore, we prepared highly purified Fos and Jun polypeptides by expressing these genes in *E. coli* (Abate *et al.*, 1990a,b). Using these proteins we reconstituted the DNA binding and transcriptional activities of the Fos–Jun complex *in vitro*. In addition, we used these proteins to screen directly cDNA expression libraries to identify other proteins capable of interacting with Fos and Jun.

To obtain high levels of Fos expression in *E. coli*, it was necessary to reconstruct the entire coding region using codons that are preferentially utilized in *E. coli*. The c-*fos*(rat) gene contains several nested sets of codons that are infrequently utilized in *E. coli* (Abate *et al.*, 1990a), and previous attempts to express Fos at high levels have been largely unsuccessful (MacConnell and Verma, 1983; Sambucetti *et*

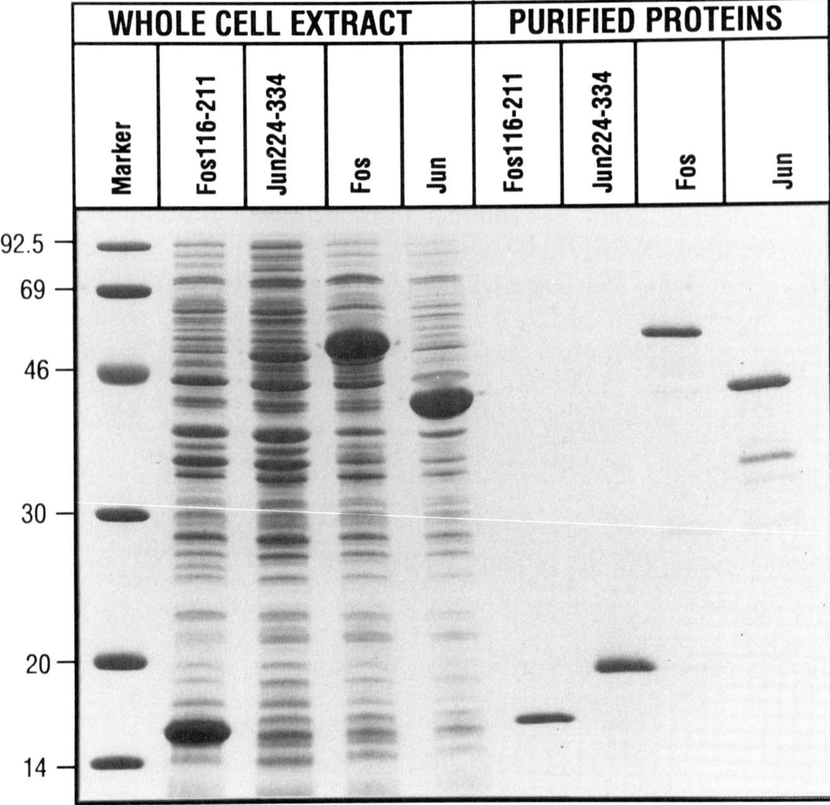

Fig. 2. Expression and purification of Fos and Jun in *E. coli*. Fos and Jun polypeptides corresponding to the full-length proteins, Fos and Jun, or truncated proteins, Fos116–211 and Jun224–334, were purified from *E. coli* cell lysates by nickel-affinity chromatography. Whole-cell lysates (10 μl) or purified proteins (2 μg) were resolved on a 13.5% SDS polyacrylamide gel and visualized by staining with Coomassie brilliant blue. Markers are molecular weight standards in kilodaltons.

al., 1986). Construction of the *fos* gene was achieved using the polymerase chain reaction to join overlapping oligonucleotides that encoded the *fos* sequence (Abate *et al.*, 1990b). Using this strategy, full-length Fos and a truncated polypeptide containing the leucine zipper and DNA-binding domain (Fos116–211) were expressed efficiently in *E. coli* (Fig. 2). In the case of Jun, high levels of expression were achieved without reconstructing the gene (Fig. 2). The Fos and Jun polypeptides were expressed as fusion proteins containing six histidine residues linked to their N-termini. Histidine fusion proteins can be rapidly and efficiently purified from *E. coli* cell lysates by affinity chromatography using a nickel chelate resin (Abate *et al.*, 1990a,b). Highly purified Fos and Jun polypeptides were obtained, using this procedure, after one pass over the nickel column (Fig. 2).

IV. A Nuclear Redox Enzyme Stimulates DNA Binding of Fos and Jun *in Vitro*

The purified Fos and Jun polypeptides efficiently formed heterodimeric complexes *in vitro* (Abate *et al.*, 1990a; Patel *et al.*, 1990). However, these proteins exhibited a low apparent affinity for DNA (Fig. 3A). This was unexpected as Fos and Jun proteins obtained by *in vitro* translation exhibited high levels of DNA-binding activity (Rauscher *et al.*, 1988c). Thus, we inferred that a component of the reticulocyte lysate contributed to the DNA-binding activity. Indeed, in the presence of the reticulocyte lysate, the *E. coli*-derived Fos and Jun polypeptides exhibited high levels of DNA-binding activity (Fig. 3A). The stimulation of DNA-binding activity was even more dramatic when a liver nuclear extract, rather than reticulocyte lysate, was included in the DNA-binding assay (Fig. 3A). These findings suggested that a cellular factor enhanced the DNA-binding activity of Fos and Jun. The stimulatory effect was observed in several different DNA-binding assays using proteins purified from mammalian sources as well as those synthesized in *E. coli*. This indicated that the stimulatory factor was of general physiological relevance rather than a peculiar feature of Fos and Jun synthesized in *E. coli*.

The stimulatory factor is a fairly ubiquitous, primarily nuclear, protein in mammalian cells (Abate *et al.*, 1990b). Its properties were investigated further using rat liver nuclear extracts as a source of activity. While the factor enhanced the affinity of Fos and Jun for the AP-1 site, it did not interact with DNA either in the presence or in the absence of Fos and Jun, suggesting that it stimulated DNA-binding activity indirectly by posttranslational modification (Abate *et al.*, 1990b). Indeed, it had several properties of a modifying enzyme. In particular, it exhibited a sharp temperature optimum, being maximally active at 37°C and inactive at 4°C (Fig. 3B). However, it did not appear to be a kinase or a phosphatase, and other posttranscriptional modifications seemed unlikely since it was active after extensive dialysis, a procedure that would remove any small-molecular-weight cofactors (Abate *et al.*, 1990a). A clue to the function of the factor was

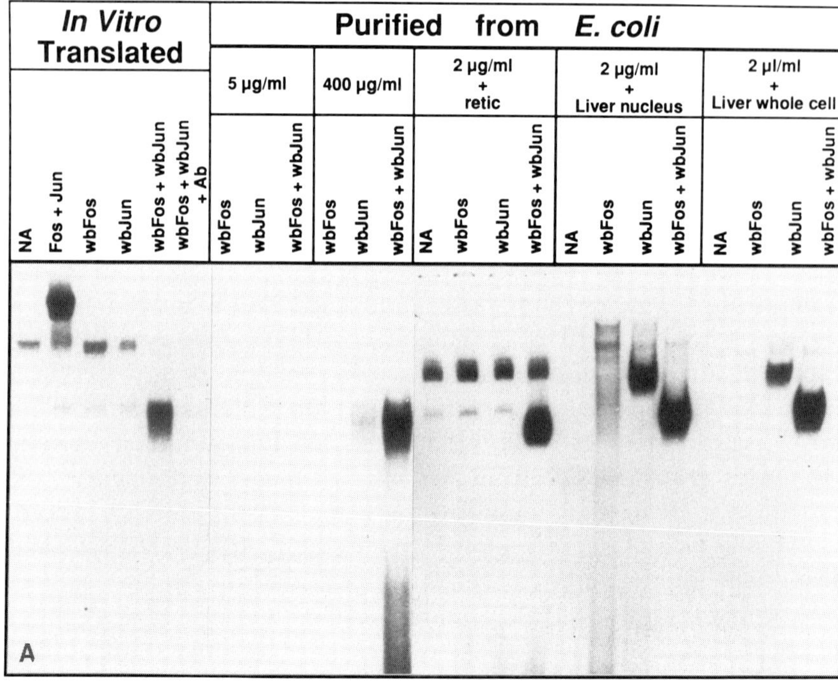

Fig. 3. DNA binding by Fos and Jun is stimulated by a cellular factor. (A) Fos and Jun, translated *in vitro* in reticulocyte lysates or purified from *E. coli,* were subjected to gel retardation assay. The *E. coli* purified proteins were assayed alone or in the presence of unprogrammed reticulocyte lysate (2 μl), liver nuclear extract (2 μg) or liver whole-cell extract (10 μg). Reprinted with permission from Abate *et al.* (1990a) *Proc. Natl. Acad. Sci. U.S.A.* **87,** 1032–1036. (B) Temperature dependence of the stimulatory factor. Fos116–211–Jun224–334 protein complexes were incubated with a radiolabelled AP-1 oligonucleotide. The protein–DNA complexes were then mixed with liver nuclear extract (2 μg) at the indicated temperatures for 0–15 min. The arrow indicates the specific protein–DNA complex. Reprinted with permission from Abate *et al.* (1990c) *Science* **249,** 1157–1161. (c) Stimulatory factor is inhibited by sulfhydryl modification. Liver nuclear extracts were untreated (lane 1), treated with the reversible sulfhydryl-modifying agent methylmethane thiosulfonate (MMTS) (lane 2), or treated with MMTS and then the agent was removed with excess DTT (lane 3). The extracts were then incubated with Fos116–211 and Jun224–334 and subjected to gel retardation assay. Reprinted with permission from Abate *et al.* (1990a) *Proc. Natl. Acad. Sci. U.S.A.* **87,** 1032–1036). (D) Stimulatory factor is activated by thioredoxin. Low concentrations of liver nuclear extract (0–0.1 μg) were incubated alone or with bovine serum albumin (BSA), thioredoxin, nicotinamide adenine dinucleotide, reduced (NADPH), or thioredoxin reductase, as indicated. The extracts were then mixed with Fos116–211 plus Jun224–334 and subjected to gel retardation assay. The arrows indicate the specific protein–DNA complexes. Reprinted with permission from Abate *et al.* (1990c) *Science* **249,** 1157–1161.

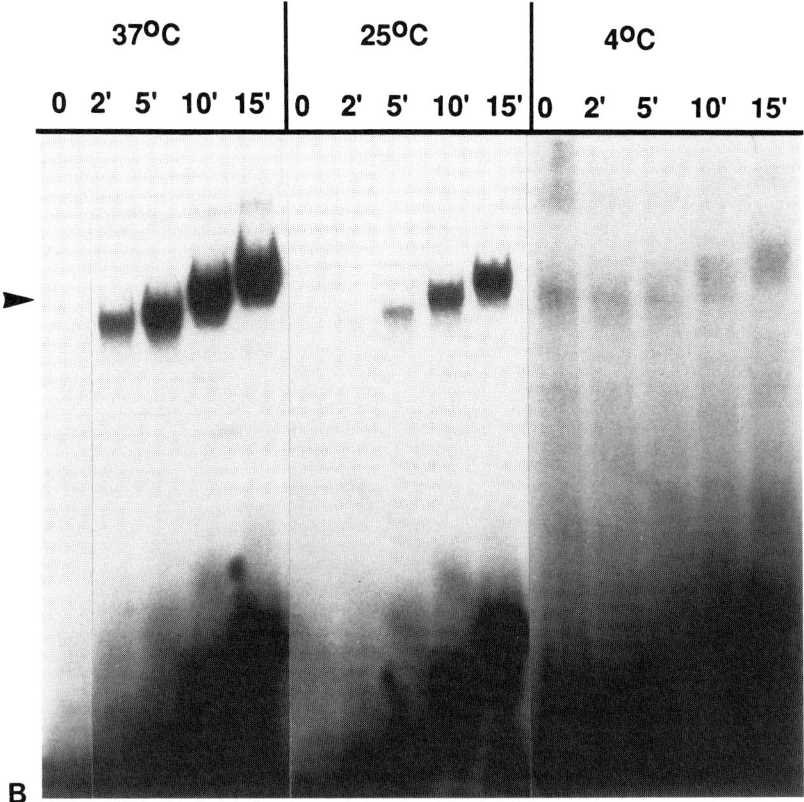

Fig. 3. *(cont.)*

the observation that its activity was abolished by treatment with sulfhydryl-modifying agents (Fig. 3C). This suggested that an active, free sulfhydryl group was required for its function. Consistent with this observation was the finding that the requirement for the stimulatory factor for Fos and Jun DNA-binding activity could be partially supplanted by the inclusion of high levels of reducing agents, such as dithiothreitol, in the DNA-binding assay (Abate *et al.*, 1990a). In addition, the stimulatory factor was activated by thioredoxin, an enzyme that catalyzes sulfhydryl reduction, whereas thioredoxin alone had no effect on Fos–Jun DNA-binding activity (Fig. 3D). Taken together, these properties suggested that a nuclear enzyme stimulated the DNA-binding activity of Fos and Jun by an oxidation–reduction mechanism. These features predicted an important role for free sulfhydryl groups in Fos and Jun for DNA-binding activity.

Fig. 3. (*cont.*)

V. A Cysteine Residue in the DNA-Binding Domain of Fos and Jun Is a Target for Regulation

The contribution of free cysteine residues in Fos and Jun to DNA-binding activity was indicated further by the sensitivity of these proteins to sulfhydryl-modifying agents (Abate *et al.*, 1990c). DNA binding of the Fos–Jun complex was reduced by the alkylating agent, *N*-ethyl maleimide (NEM); whereas incubation of the proteins with an oligonucleotide containing an AP-1 site before NEM treatment prevented inactivation (Fig. 4A). Furthermore, oxidation of Fos and Jun with the sulfhydryl-specific oxidizing agent, diamide, resulted in conversion of protein monomers to covalently cross-linked dimers (Fig. 4B). Oxidation completely abolished the DNA-binding activity of Jun homodimers and Fos–Jun heterodimers (Fig. 4C). These data

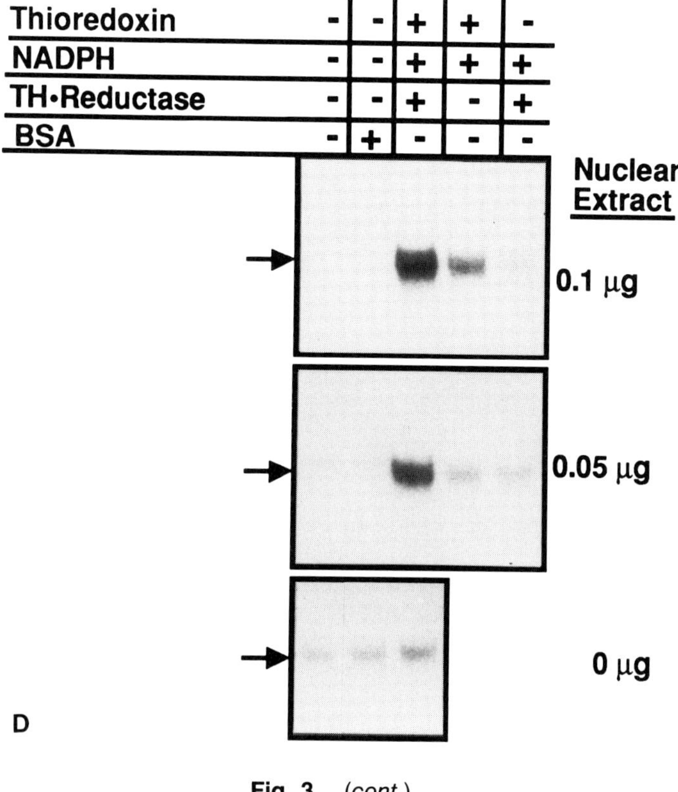

Fig. 3. (*cont.*)

demonstrate that free cysteine residues in both Fos and Jun are required for DNA binding and that these residues are in close association with DNA.

Both Fos and Jun contain a cysteine residue in the DNA-binding domain that is flanked by lysine and arginine residues. This triamino acid sequence, *lys-cys-arg,* is conserved among all members of the Fos and Jun gene families with the exception of v-Jun, the oncogenic homolog of c-*jun* (Maki *et al.,* 1987). In the context of flanking basic amino acids, cysteine residues are several orders of magnitude more reactive than cysteine residues flanked by other amino acids (Snyder *et al.,* 1981). The conservation and highly reactive nature of this cysteine indicated that it might be a candidate for regulation by a reduction–oxidation mechanism involving the stimulatory factor described in the previous section. To test this possibility, the cysteine residue in the DNA-binding domain (C1) and a cysteine residue C-

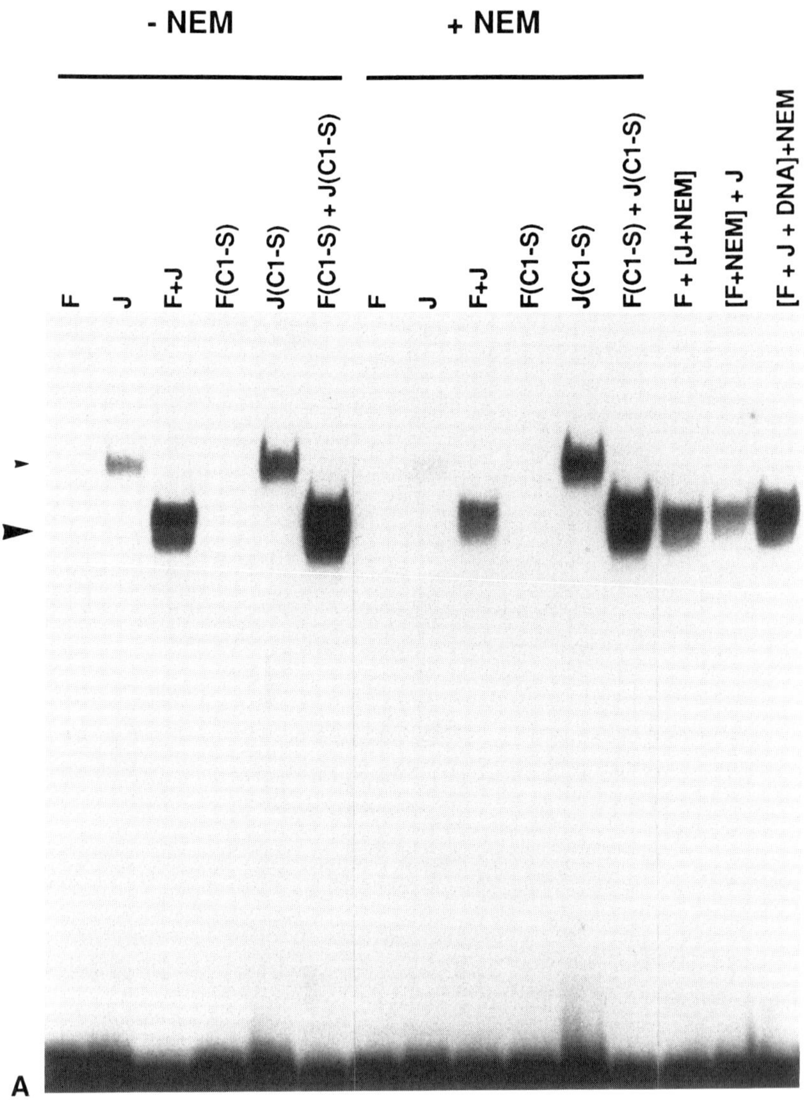

Fig. 4. (A) DNA binding by Fos and Jun is inhibited by *N*-ethyl maleimide (NEM). Fos116–211 (F) or Jun224–334 (J) were incubated in the presence (+) or absence (−) of NEM. The modified proteins were subjected to gel retardation assay. The small arrowhead indicates the position of Jun–DNA complexes, and the large arrowhead indicates the position of Fos–Jun DNA complexes. (B) Diamide oxidation of Fos and Jun converts protein momers to dimers. Fos (F) and Jun (J) were incubated in the presence (+) or absence (−) of the sulfhydryl oxidizing agent diazenedicarboxylic acid (N,N_1-dimethylamide). The proteins were resolved in a 12% nonreducing SDS polyacrylamide gel and visualized by staining with Coomassie brilliant blue. (C) Oxidation of Fos and Jun inhibits DNA binding. Fos (F) and Jun (J) protein, incubated in the presence (+) or absence (−) of diamide, were subjected to gel retardation assay. The small arrowhead indicates Jun homodimeric binding and the large arrowhead indicates the position of Fos–Jun heterodimer binding. Reprinted with permission from Abate *et al.* (1990c) *Science* **249,** 1157–1161.

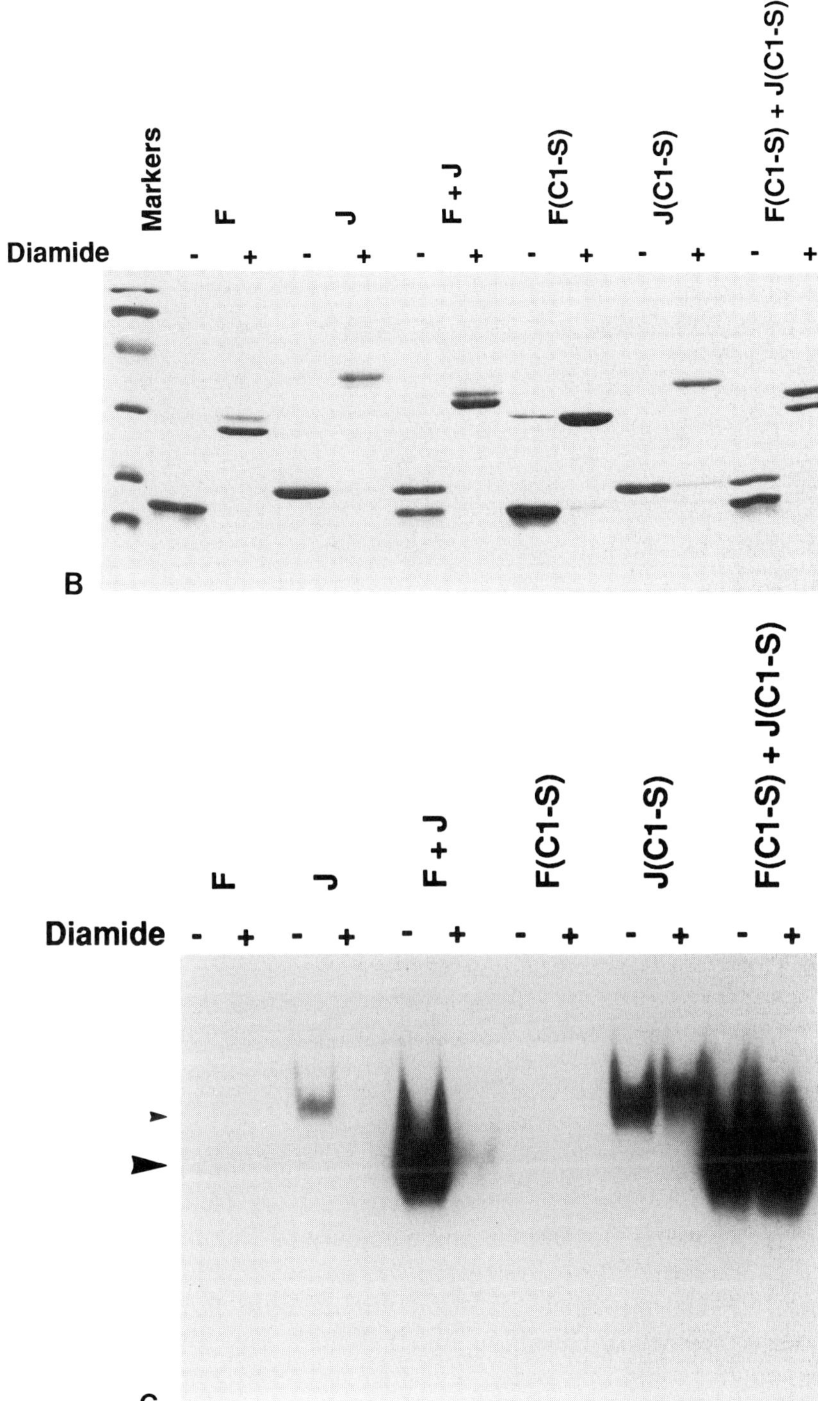
Markers
F
J
F + J
F(C1-S)
J(C1-S)
F(C1-S) + J(C1-S)
Diamide
- + - + - + - + - + - +
B
F
J
F + J
F(C1-S)
J(C1-S)
F(C1-S) + J(C1-S)
Diamide
- + - + - + - + - + - +
C

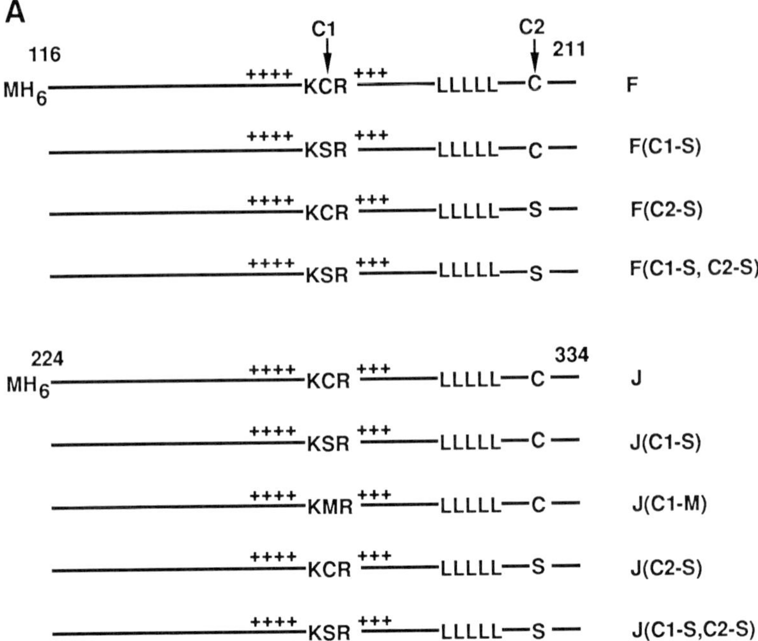

Fig. 5. (A) Mutation of critical cysteine residues in Fos and Jun enhances DNA binding. The cysteine residue (C1) in the basic region (+++) or the cysteine residue (C2) after the leucine zipper (LLLLL) in Fos (F) and Jun (J) were substituted for serine (S) or methionine (M). The specific substitutions are indicated in parentheses. (B) Fos and Jun and proteins containing the indicated substitutions were subjected to gel retardation assay in the presence of BSA (2 μg), BSA plus 5 m*M* DTT, or liver nuclear extract (2 μg). The arrow indicates the specific protein–DNA complexes. Reprinted with permission from Abate *et al.* (1990c) *Science* **249,** 1157–1161.

terminal of the leucine zipper (C2) were substituted with serine residues in both Fos and Jun (Fig. 5A). Surprisingly, Fos and Jun containing serine substitutions in the C1 position were fully active in DNA binding even in the absence of the stimulatory factor or reducing agents (Fig. 5B). The DNA-binding activity of mutated Fos and Jun that contained a C1-S substitution was not inhibited by NEM treatment (Fig. 4A). Although oxidation with diamide converted the C1-S mutated proteins to disulfide-linked dimers (Fig. 4B), these covalently-linked complexes were fully active in DNA-binding assays (Fig. 4C). These findings demonstrate that the conserved cysteine residue

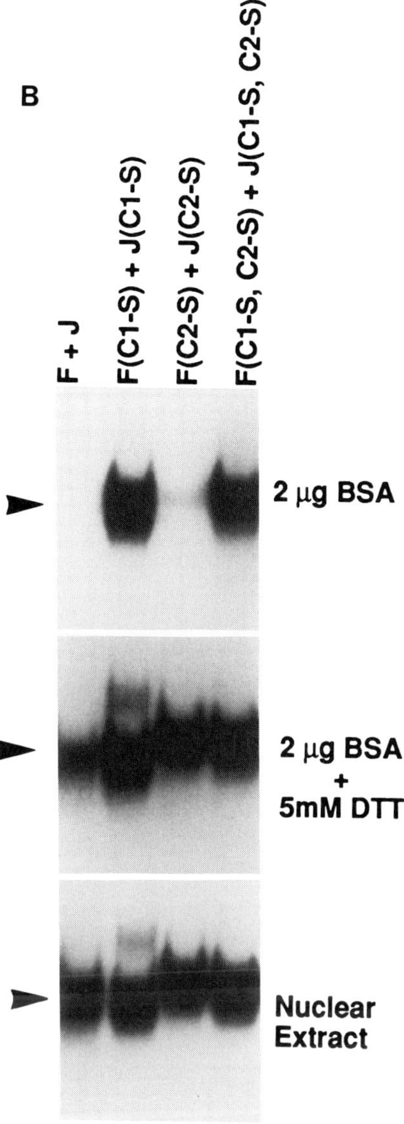

Fig. 5. *(cont.)*

in the DNA-binding domain of Fos and Jun is a target for regulation by a nuclear redox enzyme. Provocatively, v-Jun contains a serine substitution at the C1 position. This substitution may contribute to the transforming potential of *jun* by deregulation of DNA-binding activity (Abate *et al.,* 1990c).

VI. Fos and Jun Cooperate in Transcriptional Activation Via Heterologous Activation Domains

Although Fos has been widely referred to as a transcription factor, it has never been demonstrated to be such in a direct assay. The transcriptional activities of purified Fos and Jun were tested directly using HeLa cell nuclear extracts depleted of endogenous AP-1 DNA-binding activity (Abate *et al.*, 1990d). The results of these studies, presented in Fig. 6, indicate that Fos contributes directly to transcriptional activation by the Fos–Jun complex. The truncated Fos polypeptide,

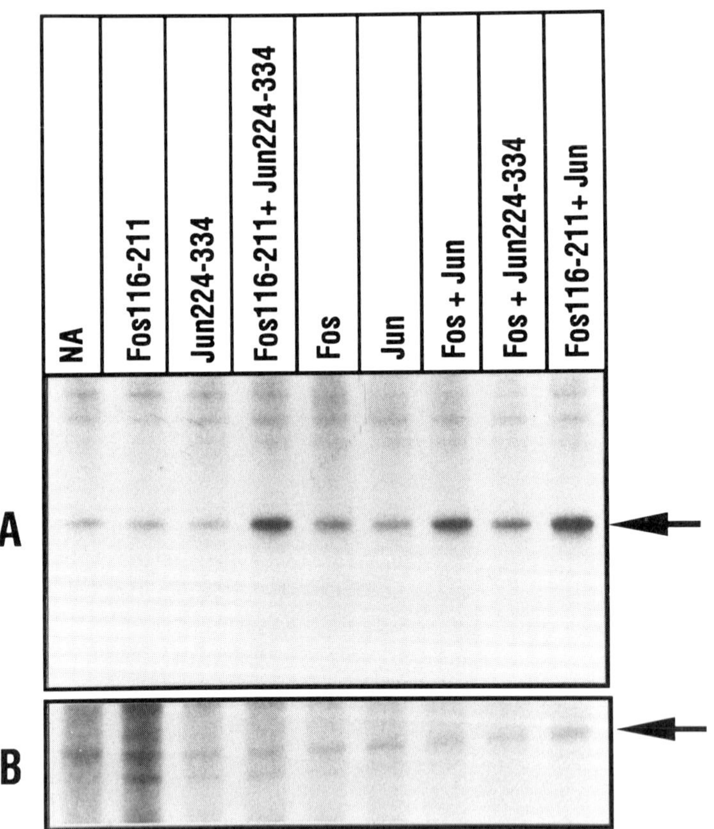

Fig. 6. Transcriptional stimulation by Fos and Jun *in vitro*. The transcriptional activities of Fos and Jun were measured using HeLa nuclear extracts as described (Abate *et al.*, 1990d). The template contained six AP-1 sites (A) or six mutated AP-1 sites (B). The arrow indicates the RNA products. Reprinted with permission from Abate *et al.* (1990d) *Mol. Cell. Biol.* **10,** 5532–5535.

Fos116–211, contains an activation domain that corresponds to a stretch of four glutamic acid residues adjacent to the DNA-binding domain. Fos116–211, in the presence of the truncated Jun protein (Jun224–334), which does not contain an activation region, produced a threefold stimulation of transcription. However, in the presence of a transcriptionally active full-length Jun protein, Fos116–211 produced a 6.5-fold stimulation of transcription (Fig. 6). Thus, domains of both Fos and Jun contribute to transcriptional activation cooperatively.

Interestingly, full-length Fos was not as active in transcriptional stimulation as the truncated Fos polypeptide. This was most evident when Fos was assayed in the presence of Jun224–334 (Fig. 6). These findings suggest that Fos contains a region(s) that exerts a negative influence on transcription. A similar property has been described for Jun (Bohman and Tjian, 1989). These regions of Fos and Jun that act negatively *in vitro* may be targets for regulation *in vivo*. It is possible that posttranslational modification of these regulatory regions could modulate the transcriptional activity of the Fos–Jun complex. Both Fos and Jun undergo extensive posttranslational modification by phosphorylation. Studies are in progress to identify the kinases that phosphorylate Fos and Jun, and to determine their contribution to the function of the Fos–Jun heterodimer.

VII. Jun Binds Cooperatively to the CRE with CRE-BP1

The previous sections described work demonstrating that Fos and Jun purified from *E. coli* efficiently formed heterodimers in solution. We reasoned that purified Jun could be used as a reagent to clone novel Jun-binding proteins. Therefore, we developed a cloning strategy to identify other leucine zipper-containing proteins capable of interacting with Fos and Jun (Macgregor *et al.*, 1990). A similar procedure has been used to clone an human immunodeficiency virus (HIV)-Tat binding protein (Nelbock *et al.*, 1990). Highly purified Fos and Jun polypeptides expressed in *E. coli* were labeled by biotinylation using biotin *N*-hydroxysuccinimide ester. The ability of the modified polypeptides to form dimers was tested in protein blot assays (Fig. 7A). In reconstitution experiments, biotinylated Jun efficiently identified plaques of bacteriophage expressing Fos (Fig. 7B). The biotinylated

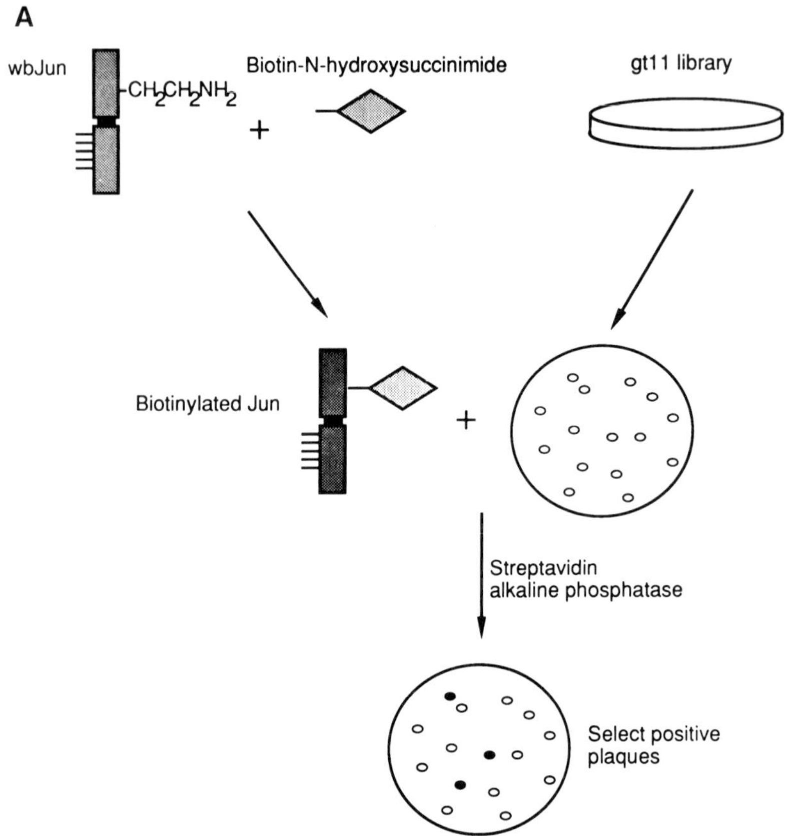

Fig. 7. (A) Protein-screening strategy. Biotin was cross-linked to wbJun primarily through lysine residues using biotin-*N*-hydroxysuccinimide ester. Approximately 1 $\mu g/ml^{-1}$ of biotinylated Jun was incubated with filters (150 mm). After washing, positive plaques were identified by treatment of the filters with streptavidin alkaline phosphatase. (B) Comparison of screening with (a) ^{32}P-labeled c-*jun* cDNA, and (b) biotinylated Jun. Plaques of phage containing Fos were readily identified by both procedures. Selected positive plaques are indicated with arrows. Reprinted with permission from Macgregor *et al.* (1990) *Oncogene* **5,** 451–458.

proteins were used to screen a λgt11 library prepared from poly(A)-containing RNA isolated from rat fibroblasts 75 min after serum stimulation (Cohen and Curran, 1988).

Screening with the biotinylated Jun polypeptide allowed isolation of several positive clones, among which clone #11 was selected for further studies. RNA transcribed from this clone was translated *in*

B

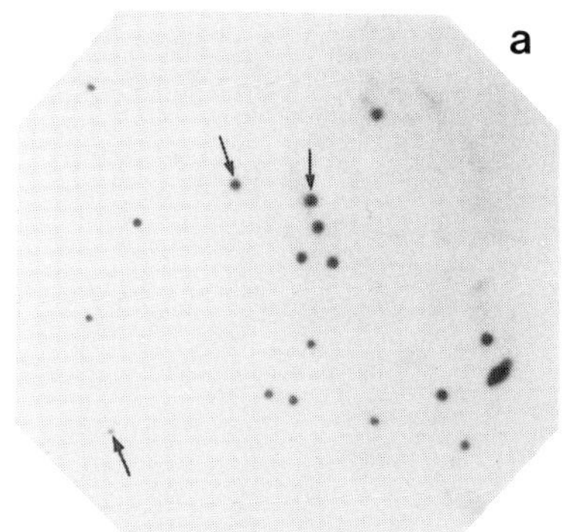

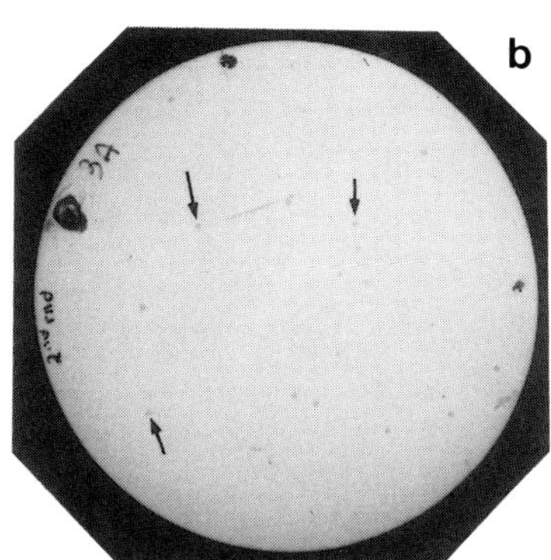

Fig. 7. (*cont.*)

vitro in rabbit reticulocyte lysates. The largest translation product obtained migrated with an apparent molecular mass of 60 kDa on sodium dodecyl sulfate (SDS)-polyacrylamide gels (Fig. 8A). This protein was not precipitated by anti-Fos or anti-Jun antibodies, indicting that clone #11 was not a Fos- or Jun-related gene. However, the protein was coimmunoprecipitated with Jun using anti-Jun antibodies (Fig. 8A). In contrast, it was not coimmunoprecipitated with Fos using anti-Fos antibodies. Nucleotide sequence analysis of clone #11 revealed that it was the rat counterpart of the cDNA encoding the cAMP-responsive element-binding protein (CRE-BP1), recently isolated by Maekawa *et al.* (1989). This clone was also isolated independently by Hai *et al.* (1989) and was referred to as ATF-2. CRE-BP1 binds specifically to the CRE DNA element as a homodimer. We investigated the effect of the heterodimer formation with Jun on DNA-binding specificity. In gel retardation assays CRE-BP1 did not bind to the AP-1 site either on its own or in the presence of Fos or Jun (Fig. 8B). In contrast, CRE-BP1 and Jun, but not Fos, formed complexes with the CRE site (Fig. 8C). Interestingly, the DNA-binding activity of the CRE-BP1-Jun heterodimer was greater than the sum of the DNA-binding activities of each protein alone, indicating that CRE-BP1 and Jun bind cooperatively to the CRE.

A similar approach was undertaken to identify novel Fos-binding proteins by direct screening with biotinylated Fos. One of the first

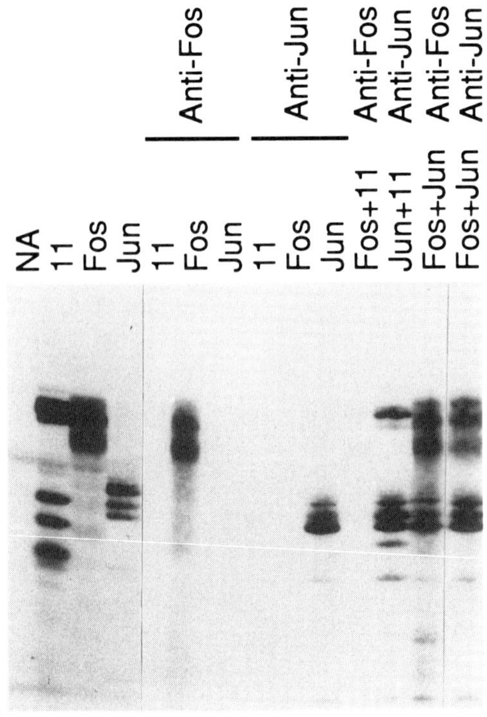

Fig. 8. The product of phage #11 dimerizes with Jun and binds to CRE sequences. (A) The protein product of positive phage #11, Fos, and Jun were expressed by *in vitro* transcription followed by translation in rabbit reticulocyte lysates. The proteins were analyzed directly or after immunoprecipitation with anti-Fos and anti-Jun antibodies on SDS polyacrylamide gels. Mixtures of Fos plus 11 and Fos plus Jun were immunoprecipitated with anti-Fos antibodies, and mixtures of Jun plus 11 and Fos plus Jun were immunoprecipitated with anti-Jun antibodies. In the case of the Fos plus 11 mixture, unlabeled Fos was used to avoid problems caused by comigration of Fos with 11. (B) Gel-shift assays were performed using reticulocyte lysates containing 11, Fos, Jun, and mixtures of Fos plus Jun, 11 plus Fos, 11 plus Jun, and 11 plus Fos plus Jun with a ^{32}P-labeled oligonucleotide containing an AP-1 site. The large arrowhead indicates the position of the Fos–Jun DNA complex, and the small arrowheads indicate the position of the Jun homodimer complex with DNA. (C) Gel-shift assays were performed using the same reticulocyte lysates described in B with an oligonucleotide containing a CRE site. In addition, mixtures of 11 plus Fos were treated with anti-Fos antibodies; mixtures of 11 plus Jun, with anti-Jun antibodies; mixtures of 11 plus Fos plus Jun, with anti-Fos antibodies; and mixtures of 11 plus Fos plus Jun, with anti-Jun antibodies. NA, no addition. An arrowhead and bracket indicate the positions of the various gel-shift activities. Reprinted with permission from Macgregor *et al.* (1990) *Oncogene* **5,** 451–458.

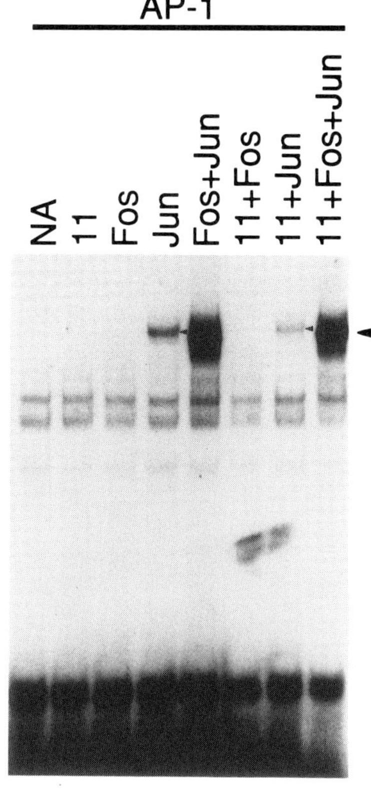

Fig. 8. (*cont.*)

clones analyzed (#F16) was shown by partial sequence analysis to be CRE-BP1. The 69-kDa protein encoded by F16, prepared by *in vitro* transcription and translation, exhibited a weak but significant level of dimerization with Fos. Since no binding was observed between Fos and the truncated version of CRE-BP1 (clone #11), this suggests that the N-terminus of CRE-BP1, which is missing in the truncated clone #11, may contribute to the formation of a heterodimeric complex between Fos and CRE-BP1. However, the heterodimer formed between Fos and full-length CRE-BP1 did not exhibit a significant level of binding to AP-1 or CRE sites (not shown). Taken together, these results demonstrate that multiple leucine-zipper protein complexes may form in stimulated cells that are capable of binding to both AP-1 and CRE sites (Fig. 1). In addition, new members of these protein complexes can be identified by a direct cloning strategy.

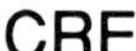

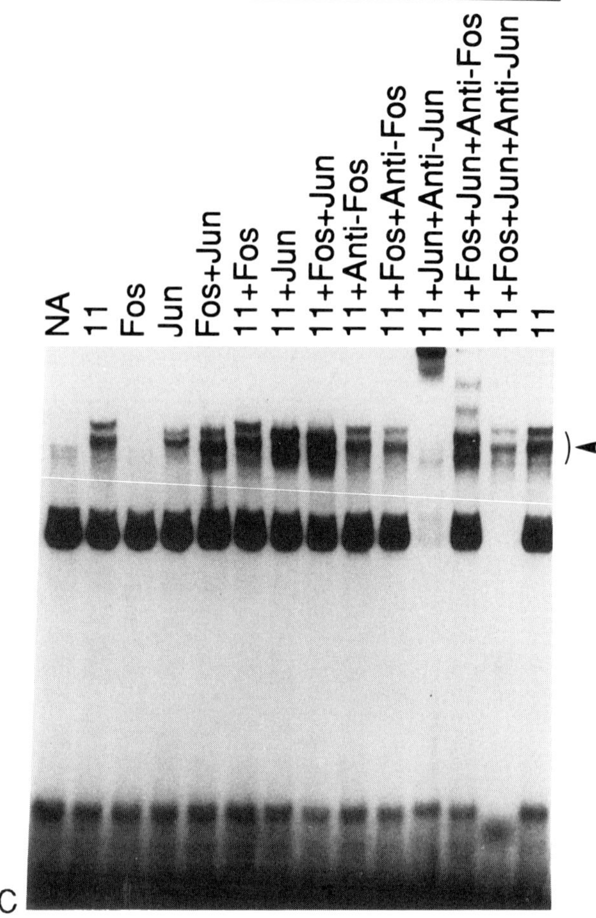

Fig. 8. (*cont.*)

VIII. Conclusions

Fos and Jun are archetypes of a set of transcription factors that function as nuclear *third-messenger* molecules in stimulus–response coupling. This set of factors is induced rapidly by a range of stimuli associated with mitogenesis, differentiation, and depolarization of neurons (Fig. 1). It is presumed that these inducible proteins act in concert with each other, and with resident transcription factors, to regulate expression of target genes that elaborate long-term phenotypic responses to environmental signals. The specificity of the response, i.e., the target genes selected for regulation, is governed by the differentiated state of the stimulated cell. There are many factors that can contribute to specificity: (1) different subsets of immediate-early genes are induced in each cell type by distinct stimuli; (2) the levels of resident transcription factors depend on the differentiated state of the stimulated cell; (3) many cellular immediate-early proteins undergo stimulus-dependent posttranslational modification; and (4) it is likely that chromatin organization influences the availability of target DNA sequences in each cell type. This level of complexity and integration of multiple signaling systems is bewildering but not necessarily unexpected. Cellular phenotypic responses are governed by the selective regulation of gene expression. To achieve the specificity required for the great diversity of such responses, gene expression must be controlled by a combinational integration of molecular signals. Our studies on the *fos* and *jun* gene families, using proteins purified from *E. coli,* have revealed some of the molecular events that contribute to stimulus-transcription coupling processes.

Fos and *jun* are members of gene families that share the leucine-zipper motif. All manner of heterodimeric complexes can be formed among these proteins, resulting in an array of transcription factor complexes capable of binding to AP-1 sites. A higher order of complexity has now been encountered as a result of the finding that Fos and Jun can dimerize with selected members of the CREB/ATF family. The CREB/ATF proteins all share the leucine-zipper motif, but their primary amino acid sequences are quite distinct, so they cannot be considered homologs of Fos or Jun. The first of these interactions between Jun and CREBP-1/ATF-2 was uncovered as a result of the development of a direct protein-screening assay (Macgregor *et al.,* 1990). Jun-CREBP-1 heterodimers bind with high affinity to CRE sites but very weakly to AP-1 sites. This is a general observation among the cross-family dimers; DNA-binding specificity is shifted toward the CRE (Hai and Curran, 1991). AP-1 (TGACTCA) and CRE (TGAGCTCA) recognition sequences are highly related and some degree of cross-specificity has been encountered. However, the heterodimerization detected among the DNA-binding proteins implies that these sites are not as distinct as previously believed. The AP-1 site has also been termed the TPA-responsive element (TRE), although this element mediates responses that are not influenced by C kinase. Similarly, the CRE has also been described as a calcium-responsive element (Sheng *et al.,* 1990). Actually, it is rather naive to imply that single DNA elements are responsible for mediating changes in gene expression by single second-messenger systems. It has long been appreciated that second-messenger signals do not operate in isolation. Furthermore, transcriptional control is generally mediated by multiple *cis*-acting sequences that are capable of interacting with several proteins. It is possible to demonstrate rather simple responses to signals using particular cell types and reiterated transcription factor recognition motifs. However, this situation is hardly ever encountered in nature, and the results of such studies may not have broad physiological significance. The ability of heterodimers of leucine zipper-containing proteins to recognize AP-1 and CRE sites implies that dimerization may control the spatial orientation of the DNA-binding domains. It is likely that the basic regions in each partner of the heterodimer recognizes a half-site in the target DNA sequence. In the CRE, the half-sites are spaced by an additional nucleotide. Thus, dimerization may result in a particular three-dimensional structure that can distinguish the many variants of AP-1 and CRE target sequences.

The identification of a novel redox mechanism that regulates the DNA-binding activity of Fos and Jun was quite unexpected. Given the many homodimeric and heterodimeric complexes capable of forming among leucine-zipper proteins, this phenomenon provides an attractive mechanism for regulation. Although redox regulation has not yet been demonstrated *in vivo,* the identification of a nuclear factor that catalyzes the reduction of Fos and Jun implies that the process is physiologically significant. At present, the exact nature and prevalence of the unusual *cys* oxidation product is unclear. It appears to represent a reversible oxidation event that occurs even under *reducing* conditions [1 m*M* dithiothreitol (DTT)]. Enzymatic reduction of this product can occur extremely rapidly. Thus, a mechanism exists whereby active protein complexes can be rendered inactive and replaced by alternatives in response to a signaling event. This process could conceivably occur within local microenvironments inside the nucleus, allowing the rapid, targeted selection of cellular immediate-early transcription factors.

References

Abate, C., and Curran, T. (1990). Encounters with Fos and Jun on the road to AP-1. *Semin. Cancer Biol.* **1**, 19–25.

Abate, C., Luk, D., Gentz, R., Rauscher, F. J., III, and Curran, T. (1990a). Expression and purification of the leucine zipper and DNA binding of Fos and Jun: Both Fos and Jun contact DNA directly. *Proc. Natl. Acad. Sci. U.S.A.* **87**, 1032–1036.

Abate, C., Luk, D., and Curran, T. (1990b). A ubiquitous nuclear protein stimulates the DNA-binding activity of Fos and Jun indirectly. *Cell Growth Differ.* (in press).

Abate, C., Patel, L., Rauscher, F. J., III, and Curran, T. (1990c). Redox regulation of Fos and Jun DNA-binding activity *in vitro*. *Science* **249**, 1157–1161.

Abate, C., Luk, D., Gagne, E., Roeder, R., and Curran, T. (1990d). Fos and Jun cooperate in transcriptional regulation via heterologous activation domains. *Mol. Cell. Biol.* **10**, 5532–5535.

Angel, P., Imagawa, M., Chiu, R., Stein, B., Imbra, R. J., Rahmsdorf, H. J., Jonat, C., Herrlich, P., and Karin, M. (1987). Phorbol ester—a TPA-modulated trans-acting factor. *Cell* **49**, 729–739.

Bohman, D., Admon, A., Turner, D. K., and Tjian, R. (1988). Transcriptional regulation by the AP-1 family of enhancer binding proteins: A nuclear target for signal transduction. *Cold Spring Harbor Symposium on Quantitative Biology* **53**, 695–700.

Bohmann, D., and Tjian, R. (1989). Biochemical analysis of transcriptional activation by Jun: Differential activity of c- and v-*jun*. *Cell* **59**, 709–717.

Bohmann, D., Bos, T. J., Admon, A., Nishimura, T., Vogt, P. K., and Tjian, R. (1987). Human protooncogene c-*jun* encodes a DNA-binding protein with structural and functional properties of transcription factor AP-1. *Science* **238**, 1386–1392.

Bos, T. J., Bohmann, D., Tsuchie, H., Tjian, R., and Vogt, P. K. (1988). Isolation and characterization of the c-*fos*(rat) cDNA and analysis of posttranslational modification *in vitro*. *Cell* **52**, 705–712.

Chiu, E., Boyle, W. J., Meek, J., Smeal, T., Hunter, T., and Karin, M. (1988). The c-*fos* protein interacts with c-*jun*/AP-1 to stimulate transcription of AP-1-responsive genes. *Cell* **54**, 541–552.

Cohen, D. R., and Curran, T. (1988). Fra-1: A serum-inducible cellular immediate-early gene that encodes for a Fos-related antigen. *Mol. Cell. Biol.* **8**, 2063–2069.

Cohen, D. R., and Curran, T. (1990). Analysis of dimerization and DNA-binding functions in Fos and Jun by domain swapping: Involvement of residues outside of the leucine-zipper basic region. *Oncogene* **5**, 929–939.

Cohen, D. R., Ferreira, P. C., Gentz, R., Franza, B. R., Jr., and Currant, T. (1989). The product of a Fos-related gene, *fra*-1, binds cooperatively to the AP-1 site with Jun: Transcription factor AP-1 is comprised of multiple protein complexes. *Genes Dev.* **3**, 173–184.

Curran, T. (1988). The Fos Oncogene. *In* "The Oncogene Handbook" (E. P. Reddy, A. M. Skalka, and T. Curran, eds.), pp. 307–325. Elsevier, Amsterdam, The Netherlands.

Curran, T., and Franza, B. R., Jr. (1988). Fos and Jun: The AP-1 connection. *Cell* **55**, 395–397.

Curran, T., and Morgan, J. I. (1987). Memories of Fos. *BioEssays* **7**, 2155–2158.

Curran, T., and Teich, N. M. (1982a). Candidate product of the FBJ murine osteosarcoma virus oncogene: Characterization of a 55,000 dalton phosphoprotein. *J. Virol.* **42,** 114–122.

Curran, T., and Teich, N. M. (1982b). Identification of a 39,000-dalton protein in cells transformed by FBJ murine osteosarcoma virus. *Virology* **116,** 221–235.

Curran, T., and Verma, I. M. (1984). The FBR murine osteosarcoma virus. I. Molecular analysis and characterization of a 75,000 *gag-fos* fusion product. *Virology* **135,** 218–228.

Curran, T., MacConnell, W. P., van Straaten, F., and Verma, I. M. (1983). Structure of the FBJ murine osteosarcoma virus genome: Molecular cloning of its associated helper virus and the cellular homolog of the v-*fos* gene from mouse and human cells. *Mol. Cell. Biol.* **3,** 914–921.

Curran, T., Miller, A. D., Zokas, L., and Verma, I. M. (1984). Viral and cellular *fos* proteins: A comparative analysis. *Cell* **36,** 259–268.

Curran, T., Rauscher, F. J., III, Cohen, D. R., and Franza, B. R., Jr. (1988). Beyond the second messenger: Oncogenes and transcription factors. *Cold Spring Harbor Symposium on Quantitative Biology* **53,** 769–777.

Curran, T., Van Beveren, C., Ling, N., and Verma, I. M. (1985). Viral and cellular Fos proteins are complexed with a 39,000-dalton cellular protein. *Mol. Cell. Biol.* **5,** 167–172.

Curran, T., Abate, C., Cohen, D. R., Macgregor, P. F., Rauscher, F. J., III, Sonnenberg, J. L., Connor, J. A., and Morgan, J. I. (1990). Inducible protooncogene transcription factors: Third messengers in the brain? CSHSQB Vol. **LV,** 225–234.

Distel, R. J., Ro, H. S., Rosen, B. S., Groves, D. L., and Spiegelman, B. M. (1987). Nucleoprotein complexes that regulate gene expression in adipocyte differentiation: Direct participation of c-*fos*. *Cell* **49,** 835–844.

Franza, B. R., Jr., Rauscher, F. J., III, Josephs, S. F., and Curran, T. (1988). The Fos complex and Fos-related antigens recognize sequence elements that contain AP-1 binding sites. *Science* **239,** 1150–1153.

Gentz, R., Rauscher, F. J., III, Abate, C., and Curran, T. (1989). Parallel association of Fos and Jun leucine zippers juxtaposes DNA-binding domains. *Science* **243,** 1695–1699.

Hai, T., Liu, F., Coukos, W. J., and Greene, M. R. (1989). Transcription factor ATF cDNA clones: An extensive family of leucine-zipper proteins able to selectively form DNA-binding heterodimers. *Genes Dev.* **3,** 2083–2090.

Hai, T., and Curran, T. (1991). Fos/Jun and ATF/CREB cross-family dimerization alters DNA-binding specificity. *Proc. Natl. Acad. Sci. U.S.A.* **88,** 3720–3724.

Halazonetis, T. D., Georgopoulos, K., Greenberg, M. E., and Leder, P. (1988). C-*jun* dimerizes with itself and with c-*fos* forming complexes of different DNA binding affinities. *Cell* **55,** 917–924.

Hill, D. E., Hope, I. A., Mackie, J. P., and Struhl, K. (1986). Saturation mutagenesis of the yeast *his* regulatory site: Requirements for transcriptional induction and for the binding of GCN4 activator protein. *Science* **234,** 451–457.

Hirai, S. I., Ryseck, R. P., Mechta, F., Bravo, R., and Yaniv, M. (1989). Characterization of JunD: A new member of the *jun* oncogene family. *EMBO J.* **8,** 1433–1439.

Hope, I. A., and Struhl, K. (1987). GCN4, a eukaryotic transcriptional activator protein binds as a dimer to target DNA. *EMBO J.* **6,** 2781–2784.

Kouzarides, T., and Ziff, E. (1988). The role of the leucine zipper in the *fos–jun* interaction. *Nature (London)* **336**, 646–651.

Kouzarides, T., and Ziff, E. (1989). Leucine zippers of *fos, jun,* and GCN4 dictate dimerization specificity and thereby control DNA binding. *Nature (London)* **340**, 568–571.

Lee, W., Haslinger, A., Karin, M., and Tjian, R. (1987a). Two factors that bind and activate the human metallothionein II_A gene *in vitro* also interact with the SV40 promoter and enhancer regions. *Nature (London)* **325**, 368–372.

Lee, W., Mitchell, P., and Tjian, R. (1987b). Purified transcription factor AP-1 interacts with TPA-inducible enhancer elements. *Cell* **49**, 741–752.

Lucibello, F. C., Neuberg, M., Hunter, J. B., Jenuwein, T., Schuermann, M., Wallich, R., Stein, R., Schonthal, H. P., Herrlich, D., and Muller, R. (1988). Transactivation of gene expression by *fos* protein: Involvement of a binding site for the transcription factor AP-1. *Oncogene* **3**, 43–51.

MacConnell, W. P., and Verma, I. M. (1983). Expression of FBJ-MSV oncogene (*fos*) product in bacterial cells. *Virology* **131**, 367–374.

Macgregor, P. F., Abate, C., and Curran, T. (1990). Direct cloning of leucine-zipper proteins: Jun binds cooperatively to the CRE with CRE-BP1. *Oncogene* **5**, 451–458.

Maekawa, T., Sakura, J., Kanei-Ishii, C., Sudo, T., Yoshimura, T., Fujisawa, J., Yoshida, M., and Ishic, S. (1989). Leucine-zipper structure of the protein CRE-BP1 binding to the cyclic AMP-responsive element in the brain. *EMBO J.* **8**, 2023–2028.

Maki, Y., Bos, T. J., Davis, C., Starbuck, M., and Vogt, P. K. (1987). Avian sarcoma virus 17 carries a new oncogene, *jun*. *Proc. Natl. Acad. Sci. U.S.A.* **84**, 2848–2852.

Matsui, M., Tokuhara, M., Konuma, Y., Nomura, N., and Ishizaki, R. (1990). Isolation of human Fos-related genes and their expression during monocyte differentiation. *Oncogene* **5**, 249–255.

Nakabeppu, Y., and Nathans, D. (1989). The basic region of Fos mediates specific DNA binding. *EMBO J.* **8**, 3833–3841.

Nakabeppu, Y., Ryder, K., and Nathans, D. (1988). DNA-binding activities of three murine *jun* proteins: Stimulation by *fos*. *Cell* **55**, 907–915.

Nelbock, P., Dillon, P. J., Perkins, A., and Rosen, C. A. (1990). A cDNA for a protein that interacts with the human immunodeficiency virus Tat transactivator. *Science* **248**, 1650–1653.

Neuberg, M., Adamkiewicz, J., Hunter, J. B., and Muller, R. (1989). Two functionally different domains in Fos are required for the sequence-specific DNA binding of the Fos/Jun protein complex. *Nature (London)* **341**, 243–245.

Nishina, H., Sato, H., Suzuki, T., Sato, M., and Iba, H. (1990). Isolation and characterization of Fra-2, an additional member of the *fos* gene family. *Proc. Natl. Acad. Sci. U.S.A.* **87**, 3619–3623.

O'Shea, E. K., Rutkowski, R., Stafford, W. F., III, and Kim, P. S. (1989). Preferential heterodimer formation by isolated leucine zipper from *fos* and *jun*. *Science* **245**, 646–648.

Patel, L., Abate, C., and Curran, T. (1990). Altered protein conformation on DNA binding by Fos and Jun. *Nature (London)* **347**, 572–575.

Rauscher, F. J., III, Cohen, D. R., Curran, T., Bos, T. J., Vogt, P. K., Bohmann, D.,

Tjian, R., and Franza, B. R., Jr. (1988a). Fos-associated protein p39 is the product of the *jun* protooncogene. *Science* **240,** 1010–1016.

Rauscher, F. J., III, Sambucetti, L. C., Curran, T., Distel, R. J., and Spiegelman, B. M. (1988b). Common DNA binding site for *fos* protein complexes and transcription factor AP-1. *Cell* **52,** 471–480.

Rauscher, F. J., III, Voulalas, P. J., Franza, B. R., Jr., and Curran, T. (1988c). Fos and Jun bind cooperatively to the AP-1 site: Reconstitution *in vitro. Genes Dev.* **2,** 1687–1699.

Reddy, E. P., Skalka, A. M., and Curran, T. (1988). "The Oncogene Handbook." Elsevier Science Publishers, Amsterdam, The Netherlands.

Renz, M., Verrier, B., Kurz, C., and Muller, R. (1987). Chromatin association and DNA-binding properties of the c-*fos* protooncogene product. *Nucleic Acids Res.* **15,** 277–294.

Ryder, K., Lanahan, A., Perez-Albuerne, E., and Nathans, D. (1988). Jun-D: A third member of the Jun gene family. *Proc. Natl. Acad. Sci. U.S.A.* **86,** 1500–1503.

Sambucetti, L. C., and Curran, T. (1986). The Fos protein complex is associated with DNA in isolated nuclei and binds to DNA cellulose. *Science* **234,** 1417–1419.

Sambucetti, L. C., Schaber, M., Kramer, R., Crowl, R., and Curran, T. (1986). The *fos* gene product undergoes extensive posttranslational modification in eukaryotic but not in prokaryotic cells. *Gene* **43,** 69–77.

Sassone-Corsi, P., Lamph, W. W., Kamps, M., and Verma, I. M. (1988). Fos-associated cellular p39 is related to nuclear transcription factor AP-1. *Cell* **54,** 553–560.

Seller, J. W., and Struhl, K. (1989). Changing *fos* oncoprotein to a *jun*-independent DNA-binding protein with GCN4 dimerization specificity by swapping "leucine zippers." *Nature (London)* **341,** 74–76.

Setoyama, C., Frunzio, R., Liau, G., Mundry, J. M., and DeCrombrugghe, B. (1986). Transcriptional activation encoded by the v-*fos* gene. *Proc. Natl. Acad. Sci. U.S.A.* **83,** 3213–3217.

Sheng, M., McFadden, G., and Greenberg, M. (1990). Membrane depolarization and calcium induce c-*fos* transcription via phosphorylation of transcription factor CREB. *Neuron* **4,** 571–587.

Snyder, G. H., Cennerazzo, M. J., Kavalis, A. J., and Field, P. (1981). Electrostatic influence of local cysteine environments on disulfide exchange kinetics. *Biochemistry* **20,** 6509–6519.

Sonnenberg, J. L., Rauscher, F. J., III, Morgan, J. I., and Curran, T. (1989). Regulation of proenkephalin by Fos and Jun. *Science* **246,** 1622–1625.

Struhl, K. (1987). The DNA-binding domains of the *jun* oncoprotein and the yeast GCN4 transcriptional activator protein are functionally homologous. *Cell* **50,** 841–846.

Turner, R., and Tjian, R. (1989). Leucine repeats and an adjacent DNA-binding domain mediate the formation of functional c-*fos* -c-*jun* heterodimers. *Science* **243,** 1689–1694.

Vogt, P. K., Bos, T. J., and Doolittle, R. F. (1987). Homology between the DNA-binding domain of the GCN4 regulatory protein of yeast and the carboxy-terminal region of a protein coded for by the oncogene *jun*. *Proc. Natl. Acad. Sci. U.S.A.* **84,** 3316–3319.

Zerial, M., Toschi, L., Ryseck, R. P., Suerman, M., Muller, R., and Bravo, R. (1989). The product of a novel growth factor-activated gene, *fos*-B, interacts with Jun proteins enhancing their DNA-binding activity. *EMBO J.* **8,** 805–813.

4

Independent Modulation of Differentiation and Proliferation in Erythroid Progenitors

HARTMUT BEUG*, GABI DOEDERLEIN†,
AND MARTIN ZENKE*

**Institute of Molecular Pathology*
Vienna, Austria

†European Molecular Biology Laboratory
Heidelberg, Germany

I. Introduction

Avian erythroblastosis virus (AEV) is an acutely leukemogenic retrovirus that induces fatal erythroleukemia in young chicks after short periods of latency. *In vitro,* AEV transforms fibroblasts as well as bone marrow cells. These *in vitro*-transformed leukemic cells represent rapidly proliferating erythroblast-like cells that are tightly arrested in an immature state of differentiation (for review see Graf and Beug, 1978, 1983). The AEV virus contains two oncogenes, a mutated version (v-*erb*B) of the epidermal growth factor receptor (EGFR) as well as a mutated, nuclear thyroid hormone receptor α (Downward *et al.,* 1984; Sap *et al.,* 1986). V-*erb*B is sufficient for transformation of fibroblasts and erythroblasts *in vivo* and *in vitro,* while the major role of v-*erb*A in erythroblast transformation is to cooperate with v-*erb*B, leading to a much more severe leukemic transformation.

The transformed phenotypes induced by the v-*erb*B oncogene in fibroblasts and hematopoietic cells (defined here as sets of *in vitro* parameters that distinguish a transformed cell from its normal counterpart) are clearly distinct. In fibroblasts, v-*erb*B causes a set of morphological changes (e.g., cell shape, cell movement, cytoskeleton), biochemical alterations (rate of hexose transport, dependence on protein growth factors), and complex changes (induction of foci or colonies in semisolid medium), but does not detectably alter the growth kinetics of fibroblasts (Royer-Pokora *et al.*, 1978; Palmieri *et al.*, 1983). In erythroid progenitors, v-*erb*B induces an abnormal type of self-renewal, characterized by a reduced expression of most, if not all erythrocyte proteins, thus preventing their accumulation in the rapidly proliferating leukemic cells. (Knight *et al.*, 1988, see also this chapter). A significant proportion of leukemic cells, however, escape this differentiation arrest and spontaneously mature into apparently normal erythrocytes (Beug *et al.*, 1985; Kahn *et al.*, 1986). In addition, v-*erb*B renders erythroid progenitors independent of the erythroid growth/differentiation hormone erythropoietin (EPO; Beug *et al.*, 1985; Kowenz *et al.*, 1987). This abrogation of EPO dependence by v-*erb*B could be separated from self-renewal induction by this oncogene since human c-*erb*B/EGFR induced the latter but not the former effect in erythroblasts when activated by ligand (EGF), whereas a 31-amino acid C-terminal deletion mutant of c-*erb*B/EGFR was able to cause both changes (Khazaie *et al.*, 1988).

The v-*erb*A oncogene, a mutant thyroid hormone receptor α (TRα) has lost its ability to up-regulate gene expression in response to ligand but has retained its activity as a repressor in absence of ligand (Damm *et al.*, 1989; Sap *et al.*, 1989). V-*erb*A has only subtle effects on fibroblasts. It causes a moderate increase in growth rate, *in vitro* life span, and ability to form agar colonies in cultured fibroblasts, and appears to affect matrix protein production in fibroblasts implanted into the chorioallantoic membrane of chick embryos (Gandrillon *et al.*, 1987). In erythroid cells, v-*erb*A again affects the differentiation phenotype, albeit in a fashion very different from that of v-*erb*B. While v-*erb*B as well as other kinase oncogenes (*sea, src,* etc.) seem to reduce but not totally prevent expression of a large number of erythrocyte proteins (Knight *et al.*, 1988), v-*erb*A probably acts as a specific and effective repressor of a small subset of erythrocyte genes. Three of these genes have been identified so far, e.g., carbonic anhydrase II (CA II), erythrocyte anion transporter (Band 3), and δ-aminolevulinic synthethase (Ala S), the first enzyme in heme biosynthesis (Zenke *et al.*, 1988, 1990). This specific repression of some but not all erythroid genes at least contributes to the phenotype caused by v-*erb* A in erythroblasts (i.e., partially mature erythroid cells with some aberrant features), which clearly differs from that induced by v-*erb*B and related oncogenes (Schroeder *et al.*, 1990). Studies with certain mutant v-*erb*A proteins suggest that v-*erb*A might also increase the growth rate of kinase-oncogene transformed erythroblasts (Forrest *et al.,* 1990).

Thus, the described features of leukemic transformation by AEV seem to predominantly involve complex alterations of the *differentiation program* of infected erythroid progenitors. This notion is somewhat difficult to reconcile with currently prevailing ideas that neoplastic transformation is the consequence of aberrant *proliferation* control, brought about by activation or loss of genes (protooncogenes) that are part of the complex network positively or negatively controlling the cell cycle (Alberts *et al.,* 1983; Kahn and Graf, 1986). A possible reason for such an (obviously too simple) model is another textbook hypothesis stating that terminal differentiation and proliferation are mutually exclusive, i.e., that a cell has to leave the cell cycle in order to differentiate and that maintenance of a proliferative state would automatically prevent or slow down maturation (Alberts *et al.,* 1983; Alema and Tato, 1987). Whereas such a process is undoubtedly going on during normal maturation of many cell types (almost all terminally differentiated cells are stationary) and may also be true for certain oncogenes (La Rocca *et al.,* 1989), it is less clear whether there is a mechanistic relationship (i.e., increased proliferation-blocking differentiation) that would also be evident in abnormal situations (e.g., transformed cells).

Differentiating erythroid precursors are a particularly attractive system to use for a closer look at this question since these cells differentiate and proliferate simultaneously (Alberts *et al.,* 1983). It is clear from many studies that the erythroid progenitor referred to as CFU-E (colony-forming unit, erythroid) gradually accumulates hemoglobin and other erythrocyte proteins while it undergoes four to six cell divisions, the cells withdrawing from cell cycle only as fully mature cells. The availability of two oncogenes (v-*erb*A and v-*erb*B) that affect this differentiation program in a clearly distinct fashion, as well as the possibility of separately turning these oncogenes on or off at will (Beug *et al.,* 1982; Beug and Hayman, 1984; Zenke *et al.,* 1988) prompted us to question whether proliferation and differentiation in this system are two separate genetic programs that can be independently altered by oncogenes or whether the change of one program would affect the other one.

In this chapter, some (in part preliminary) results obtained with two different types of conditional kinase oncogenes (ts *sea*/ts *erb*B regulated by temperature; human c-*erb* B/EGFR regulated by EGF; Knight *et al.,* 1988; Khazaie *et al.,* 1988) as well as with v-*erb*A functionally turned on or off by medium pH (Zenke *et al.*, 1988) will be discussed. Our results suggest that under certain conditions both oncogenes can alter the differentiation program without drastically changing cell-proliferation properties. In addition, it will be demonstrated that under certain experimental conditions, a complete arrest of the cell cycle in erythroid progenitors does not detectably alter their ability to terminally differentiate into erythrocytes.

II. Results

A. Conditional Kinase Oncogenes Alter the Erythroid Differentiation Program Independent of Their Effects on Proliferation

1. Reversibility of Early Erythroid Differentiation

Overexpression of the normal human EGFR in erythroid progenitors leads to the outgrowth of transformed erythroblasts in response to ligand (EGF). Simple withdrawal of EGF is sufficient to abolish the transformed phenotype and induce normal, EPO-dependent erythroid differentiation (Khazaie *et al.*, 1988). It was thus of interest to compare the growth properties of EGFR-expressing erythroblasts growing in EGF (thus in a differentiation-blocked state) or after switch to EPO-containing medium (leading to differentiation induction). In these experiments, EGFR-ts-*myb* erythroblasts were used instead of EGFR erythroblasts because of the much prolonged *in vitro* life span of the former (see Section IV, "Materials and Methods"; Beug *et al.*, unpublished). In addition, cells were cultivated in EPO-containing medium for periods insufficient to cause commitment of the majority of the cells (22 hr; Beug *et al.*, 1982). They were then switched back to EGF-containing medium, and their proliferation and differentiation properties analyzed. As shown in Fig. 1A, the proliferation kinetics of cells grown in EGF for 72 hr or switched to EPO-containing medium after 22 hr were virtually indistinguishable. As expected, the cells switched to EPO differentiated into late reticulocytes with normal kinetics (see Fig. 1B), whereas the EGF-grown cells stayed immature (Fig. 1A). Interestingly, the opposite switch (EPO to EGF after 22 hr) caused a decrease in growth rate and ^{3}H-thymidine incorporation rather than the expected increase (Fig. 1B, C). This may be owing to the fact that no reversion of the partially mature state obtained after 22 hr was observed after switch from EPO

A

EGF
continuously
EGF 22 hours,
then EPO
Ery
LR
ER
Ebl
Cumulative cell number (x 10 6)
1000
100
10
0
20
40
60
80
hours in culture

B

EPO
continuously
EPO 22 hours,
then EGF
Ery
LR
ER
Ebl
Cumulative cell number (x 10 6)
1000
100
10
0
20
40
60
80
hours in culture

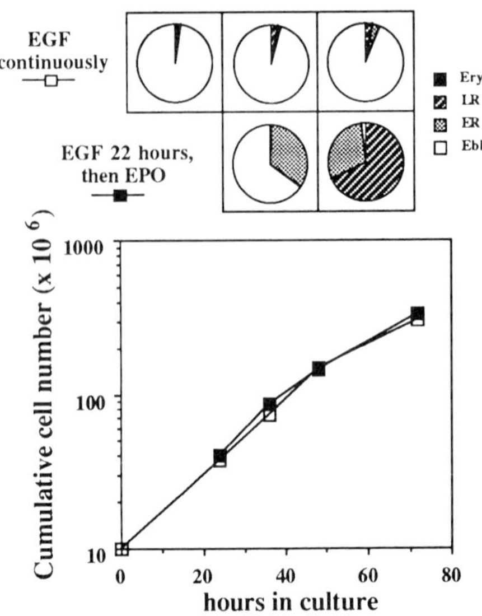

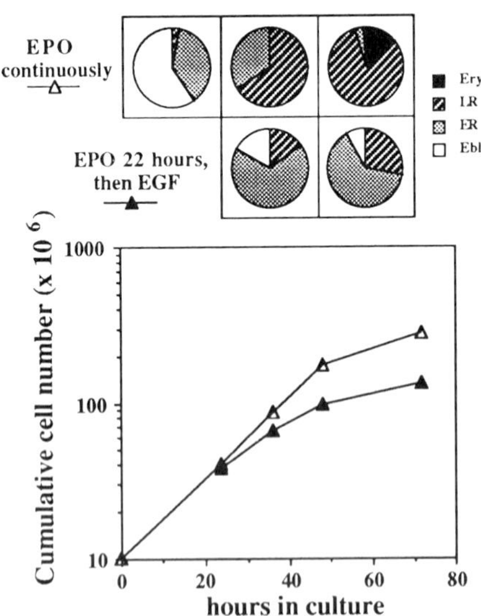

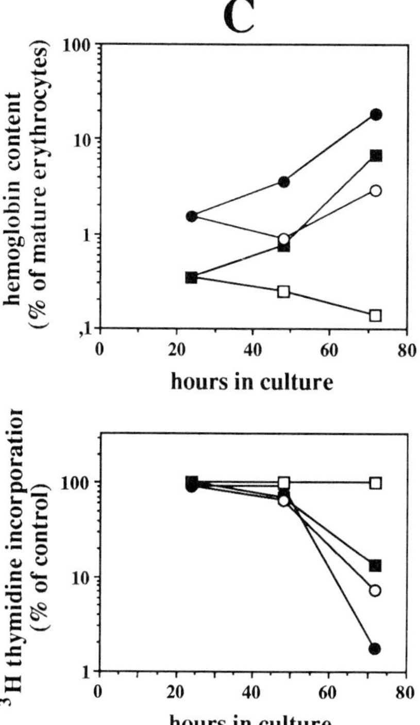

Fig. 1. Proliferation and differentiation of EGFR-ts v-*myb* erythroblasts switched between differentiation-inducing (EPO) and transformation-inducing (EGF) conditons. (A, B) Cells were grown at 42°C in EGF-containing (20 μg/ml) differentiation medium (A, open squares) or EPO-containing medium (B, open triangles), and cell numbers were determined at the times indicated. After 22, 48, and 72 hr (upper rows of pie diagrams, from left to right) cells were cytocentrifuged onto slides and stained with neutral benzidine. The percentages of erythroblasts (Ebl, white areas), early reticulocytes (ER, dotted areas), late reticulocytes (LR, hatched areas), and erythrocytes (Ery, black areas) were determined as described (Beug *et al.,* 1982). Alternatively, cells grown in EGF or EPO for 22 hr were switched to EPO- (solid squares) or EGF-containing media (solid triangles), respectively, and analyzed for proliferation and differentiation (lower rows of pie diagrams) as above. (C) Cells grown in EGF (open squares), EPO (solid circles) and switched from EGF to EPO (solid squares) or from EPO to EGF (open circles) as described were analyzed for hemoglobin content (upper panel) or ^{3}H-thymidine incorporation (lower panel) as described in Section IV, Materials and Methods.

to EGF; rather, the cells continued to mature with grossly slowed down kinetics (Fig. 1B). This idea was confirmed by measuring the hemoglobin content of the different cell populations. To our surprise, the hemoglobin content of the cells switched from EPO to EGF re mained roughly constant at an intermediate level (Fig. 1C). As expected, the cells grown in or switched to EPO accumulated hemoglobin (Hb) rapidly, whereas the EGF-grown transformed cells failed to accumulate Hb (Fig. 1C).

Next, we tried to analyze how the switch from EPO to EGF would affect the expression of erythroid-specific genes. For this, EGFR-ts-*myb* erythroblasts were grown for 16 hr at 42°C in medium containing either EGF or EPO, washed, and grown in medium containing the other hormone for increasing lengths of time. The expression levels of CA II, band 3, α-globin, and (as a control) c-*myb* were then determined by slot-blot analysis using total RNA prepared from the respective cell populations (Zenke *et al.*, 1990, Fig. 2).

The switch from EGF- to EPO-containing medium showed the result expected from earlier studies using ts v-*sea* erythroblasts (Knight *et al.*, 1988). While CA II expression (abnormally elevated in transformed cells, Knight *et al.*, 1988) rapidly decreased, band 3 and globin messages increased after 16 hr, whereas only a slight increase was seen after 6 hr Fig. 2. In line with their differentiation phenotype and hemoglobin content, EGFR-ts-*myb* erythroblasts switched from EPO- to EGF-containing medium failed to down-regulate band 3 and α-globin mRNA levels within the experimental period (16 hr). In contrast, a rapid up-regulation of CA II message was seen, indicating the restoration of tyrosine kinase-induced abnormal expression of this gene (Knight *et al.*, 1988).

2. *Effect of "Partially Active" Kinase Oncogenes on Proliferation and Differentation of Erythroid Cells*

The availability of erythroid cells transformed by ligand-activated EGFR allowed us to study how this tyrosine kinase *oncogene* would affect proliferation and differentiation of erythroblasts at different levels of kinase activity induced by different concentrations of ligand (EGF). Whereas the proliferation rate (Fig. 3A) and rate of thymidine incorporation per 10^5 viable cells (Fig. 3B) showed only a moderate decline with decreasing EGF concentrations, erythroid differentiation was strongly affected by EGF concentration (Fig. 3C). Formation of mature cells was already significantly induced at 4 and 1 μg/ml EGF;

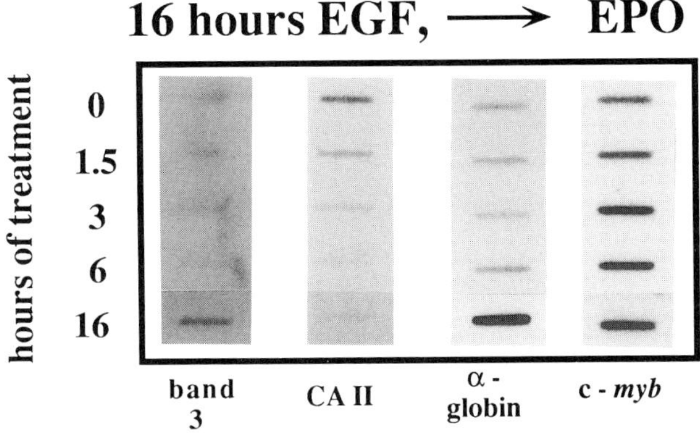

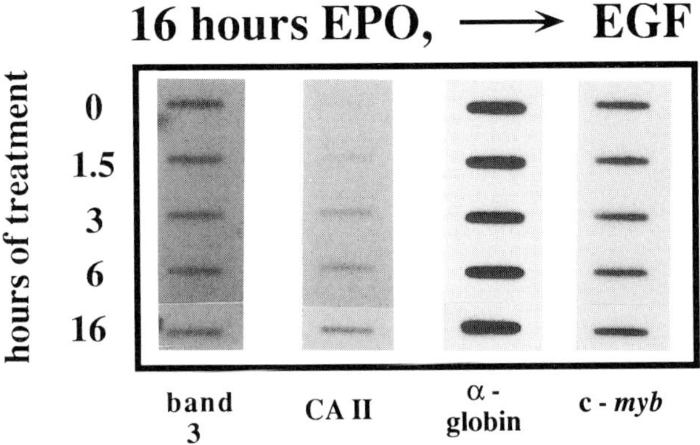

Fig. 2. Expression of erythrocyte-specific genes in EGFR-ts v-*myb* erythroblasts switched between transformation- and differentiation-inducing conditions. Cells switched between EGF- and EPO-containing media (see legend of Fig. 1) were harvested after the times indicated (hours of treatment) and analyzed for expression of erythrocyte-specific genes and c-*myb* (as a control) by the slot-blot technique as described in Section IV, Materials and Methods.

the speed of maturation was inversely related to EGF concentration (Fig. 3C).

A second, independent approach to studying the effect of a kinase oncogene at different activity states on proliferation and differentiation of erythroblasts consisted of inducing the differentiation of ts v-*sea*-transformed erythroblasts at different, carefully controlled temperatures. As will be described in detail elsewhere, the cells were grown in small, water-jacketed CO_2-incubators allowing maintainance of temperatures between 30 and 45°C with an accuracy of 0.1 to 0.05°C. Pilot experiments showed that cells were fully transformed

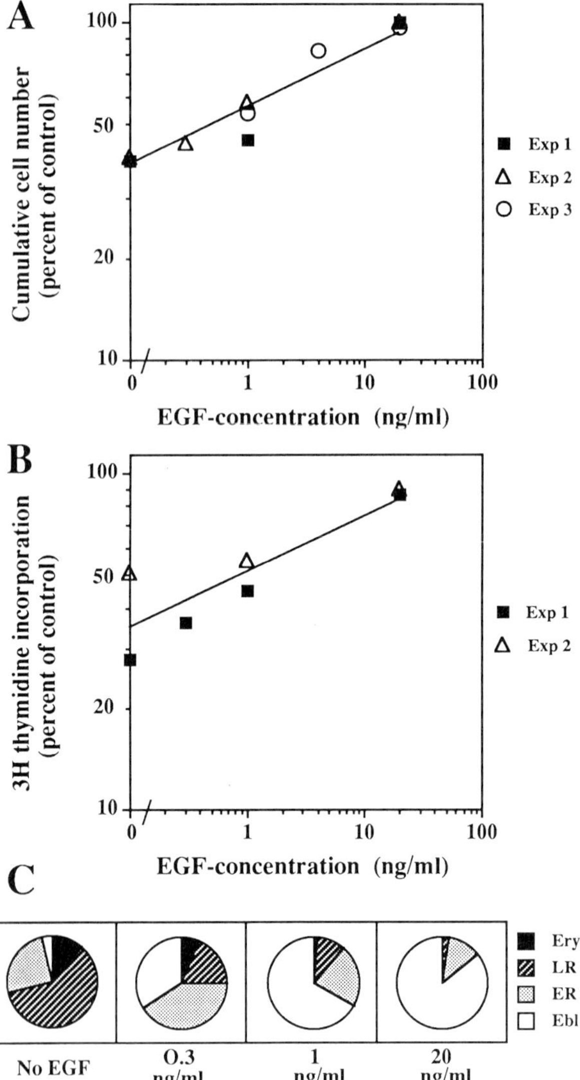

Fig. 3. Modulation of c-*erb*B/EGFR tyrosine kinase activity in differentiating erythroblasts. C-*erb*B/EGFR erythroblasts (Khazaie *et al.*, 1988) were cultivated in EPO-containing differentiation media in presence of the EGF-concentrations indicated and analyzed for cumulative cell numbers (A) and ^{3}H-thymidine incorporation (B) after 2 days and for differentiation by neutral benzidine staining after 3 days (C); see legend of Fig. 1.

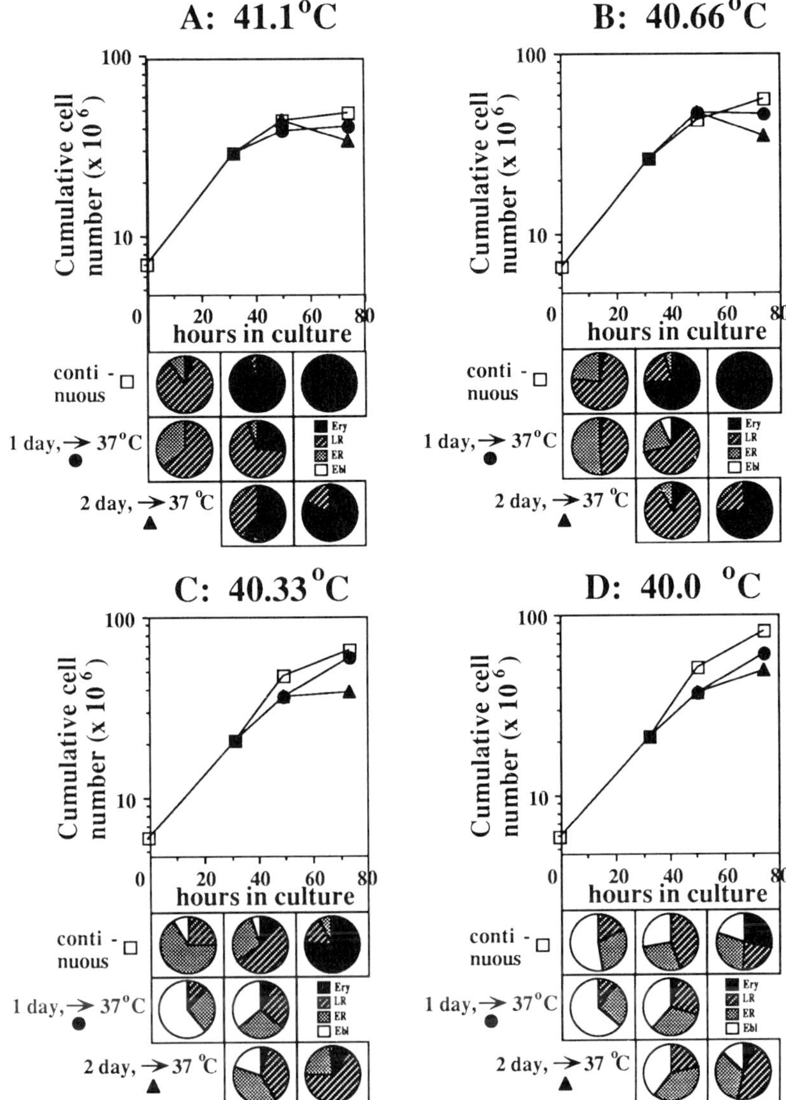

Fig. 4. Modulation of ts v-*sea* oncogene activity: Proliferation, differentiation, and commitment of ts v-*sea* erythroblasts at temperatures between permissive and nonpermissive conditions. (A, B, C, D) upper panels: Ts v-*sea* erythroblasts were cultivated at four different temperatures between permissive (39.5°C) and nonpermissive temperature (41.3°C) for the times indicated, and cumulative cell numbers were determined (open squares). Alternatively, cells were shifted back to 37°C after incubation at the respective temperatures for 24 hr (closed circles) or 48 hr (closed triangles) and counted at the times indicated. (A, B, C, D) lower panels: Differentiation was analyzed by neutral benzidine staining of cytospin preparations (see legend to Fig. 1) in all cell preparations after 50 hr (left pie diagrams), 74 hr (middle pie diagrams), and 96 hr of culture (right pie diagrams).

at 39.5°C, whereas they differentiated with normal kinetics at 41.2°C. We therefore analyzed the proliferation and differentiation kinetics of ts v-*sea* erythroblasts at four intermediate temperatures (Fig. 4). To determine the extent and speed of commitment to erythroid differentiation (Beug *et al.*, 1982), aliquots of the cells preparations were shifted back to 37°C after 1 and 2 days.

The results clearly demonstrate that the growth rate of ts v-*sea* erythroblasts was hardly altered by temperature during the first 48 hr, whereas the speed of maturation was drastically affected by temperature. Thus, >75% mature cells (LR + E, see Material and Methods) were obtained after 50 hr at 41.1°C; Fig. 4A), whereas it took 74 hr at 40.66°C (Fig. 4B) and 96 hr at 40.33°C (Fig. 4C) to reach this state of maturation. At 40.0°C, only 50% LR + E were obtained after 96 hr. Consistent with the notion that proliferation arrest of differentiating red cell precursors is a late event, proliferation rate started to decrease between 31 and 50 hr only at 41.1°C, whereas this decrease occurred between 50 and 74 hr at 40.66°C and 40.33°C and not at all at 40.0°C. Thus, the gradual loss of proliferative capacity seems to occur at the stage of late reticulocytes (characterized by the beginning loss of organelles like ribosomes and mitochondria; Beug *et al.*, 1982).

The activity of the kinase also seemed to influence the length of the commitment period. At 41.1°C, commitment was essentially complete after 24 hr since >95% mature cells were obtained from cultures shifted back to 37°C after that period (Fig. 4A and data not shown). At 40.66°C, commitment was incomplete after 24 hr, but complete after 48 hr (Fig. 4B). At 40.33°C, 48 hr was sufficient for almost complete commitment, whereas at 40.0°C, only part of the cells became committed even after 48 hr (Fig. 4C, D and data not shown).

In a final experiment, proliferation and differentiation kinetics of ts v-*sea*-erythroblasts cultivated at different temperatures (see previous paragraphs) were compared in presence and absence of EPO. This erythroid growth factor was shown earlier to regulate survival and proliferation of erythroid progenitors without apparently altering their differentiation program (Kowenz *et al.*, 1987; Knight *et al.*, 1988). The results shown in Table I demonstrate that at all temperatures, proliferation was much slower in the absence than in the presence of EPO (as evidenced by longer doubling times and lower cumulative cell numbers in absence of the hormone). In contrast, the speed and

TABLE I

Proliferation and Differentiation of ts-v-sea Erythroblasts in the Presence and Absence of Erythropoietin (EPO)

	+EPO				−EPO			
		E + LR[a] (%)				E + LR (%)		
Temperature (°C)	Doubling time (hr)	50 hr[b]	74 hr	96 hr	Doubling time (hr)	50 hr	74 hr	96 hr
41.1	15 (48)[c]	91	100	100	22 (27)	84	98	100
40.66	15.5 (48)	77	96	100	22.5 (29)	73	93	100
40.33	16 (66)	25	65	93	26 (33)	10	51	87
40.0	16 (79)	17	44	51	23 (39)	8	25	76

[a] E + LR, erythrocytes and late reticulocytes; Beug *et al.* (1982).
[b] 50 hr, 50 hr after shift to the respective temperature.
[c] Numerals in brackets, cumulative cell number accrued $\times 10^{-6}$.

extent of erythroid differentiation occurring in the absence of EPO was hardly distinguishable from that obtained in presence of the hormone (Table I). Thus, changing the growth rate of differentiating erythroid progenitors did not seem to markedly affect the kinetics of differentiation, although this latter parameter was itself strongly modulated by different activity levels of the ts v-*sea* oncogene.

B. The Ability of the v-*erb*A Oncogene to Arrest Erythroid Differentiation Can Be Gradually Turned On or Off by Specific Changes in Culture Conditions

As described above, the possibility of altering the bioactivity of an oncogene in a gradual fashion (e.g., activation of c-*erb*B/EGFR by increasing concentrations of EGF or altering the activity of ts v-*sea* by cultivating the cells at different, carefully controlled temperatures) turned out to be a useful tool for dissecting the pleiotropic effects of oncogenes on proliferation and differentiation of erythroblasts. As published earlier, the bioactivity of the v-*erb*A oncogene could be turned off by cultivating the cells in media of alkaline pH (pH 8.1) generated by partial replacement of NaCl by $NaHCO_3$ (Beug *et al.*, 1982; Zenke *et al.*, 1988). To determine whether this approach could

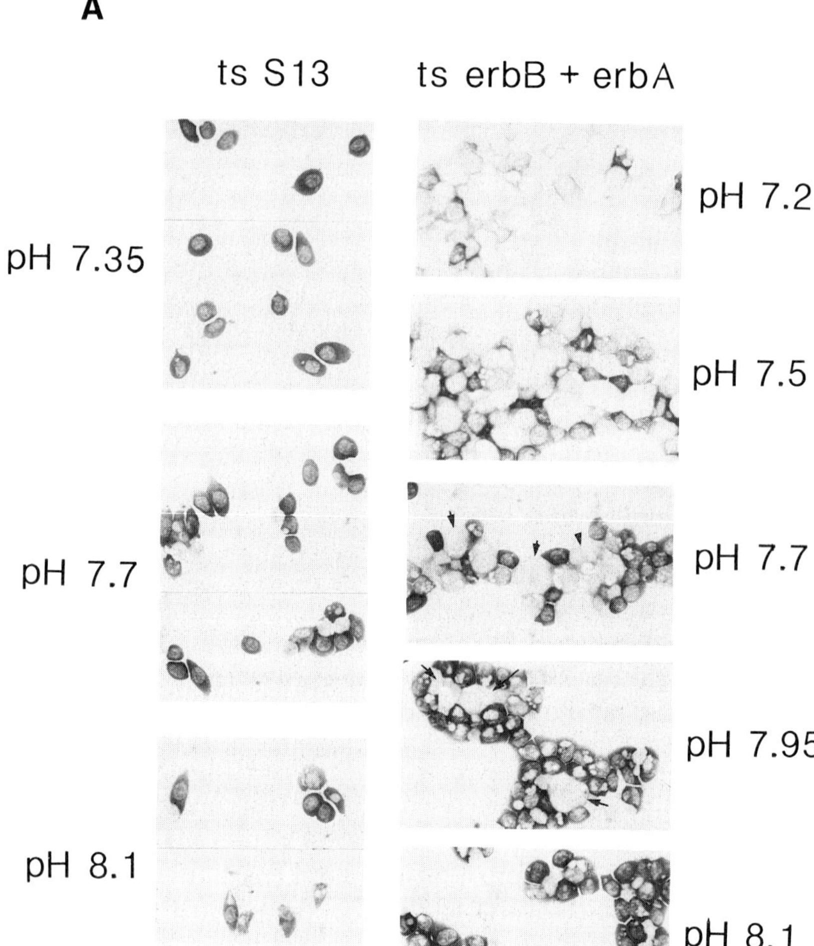

Fig. 5. Proliferation and differentiation of v-*erb*A/ts v-*erb*B erythroblasts in which the activity of v-erbA is modified by medium pH. (A) Erythroblasts containing v-*erb*A (ts *erb*B + *erb*A; ts 167 AEV erythroblasts, clone E3; Zenke *et al.*, 1988) or lacking v-*erb*A (ts S 13; ts *sea* erythroblasts clone A 4) were cultivated at 42°C in media of the indicated pH values for 3 days, cytocentrifuged onto slides, stained with neutral benzidine and histochemical dyes, and photographed under blue light to reveal staining for hemoglobin (Beug *et al.*, 1982). Right panels: Note the increasing appearance of partially mature (gray) and mature (black, oval) ts 167 AEV cells in media of increasing pH. Some erythroblasts prevailing at pH 7.7 and 7.95 are indicated by arrows. Left panels: Note that the ts v-*sea* (ts S 13) cells exhibit a mature phenotype at all pH values tested. (B) The same cell clones as in A (containing or lacking v-*erb*A) were seeded into 96 well plates in media of

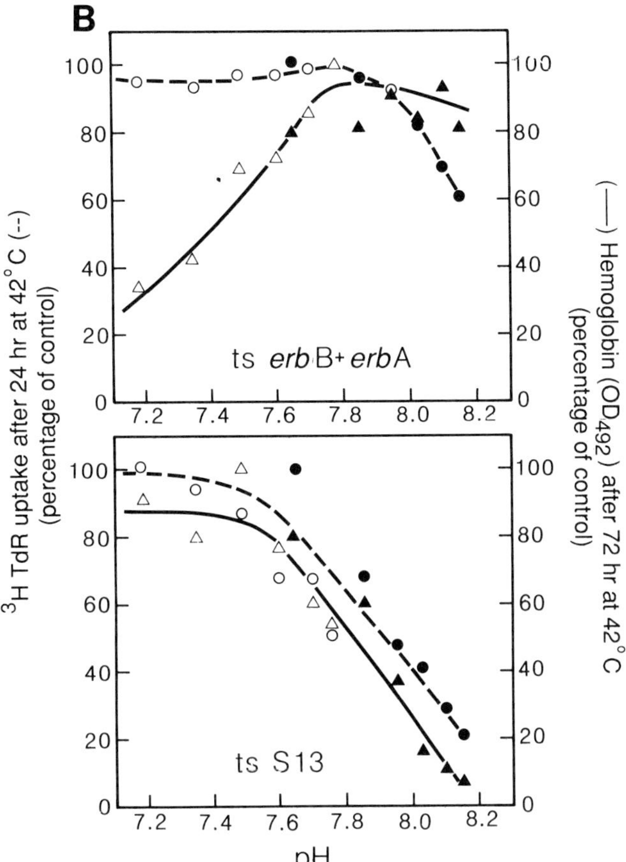

different pH (see Section IV, Materials and Methods) and analyzed for ^{3}H-thymidine incorporation (^{3}H TdR uptake, circles) and hemoglobin (OD 492) after 24 hr and 72 hr at 42°C, respectively, using the assays described in Kowenz *et al.* (1987). The actual pH values of the different media were determined in control medium samples as described in Beug and Graf (1977). Open symbols, cultures kept at 10% CO_2; closed symbols, cultures kept at 2% CO_2; respectively.

be used to gradually change the bioactivity of the v-*erb*A oncogene (i.e., its ability to arrest differentiation), ts 167 AEV (ts *erb*B + v-*erb*A; Palmieri *et al.*, 1982) erythroblasts and, as a control, ts v-*sea* erythroblasts were induced to differentate at 42°C, using media in which the pH/$NaHCO_3$ concentration was varied gradually (see Section IV, Kahn *et al.*, 1986). The cells were then analyzed for their proliferation capacity by measuring ^{3}H-thymidine incorporation and for their differentiation program by neutral benzidine staining (Beug *et al.,* 1982) and quantitative hemoglobin analysis (Kowenz *et al.,* 1987).

In ts 167 AEV cells, the extent of erythroid differentiation occuring within 3 to 4 d was completely dependent on medium pH (Fig. 5A). Whereas cells remained essentially immature at pH 7.2, about 20%, 50%, 80% and >95% of the cells differentiated at pH 7.5, 7.7, 7.95, and 8.1, respectively. No such pH dependence of differentiation was seen in ts v-*sea* erythroblasts devoid of v-*erb*A (Fig. 5A), suggesting that the pH dependence of ts 167 AEV erythroblasts was in fact the result of gradual inactivation of v-*erb*A activity by media of increasing pH.

The notion that gradual v-*erb*A inactivation by medium pH led to a progressive induction of erythroid differentiation in ts 167 AEV erythroblasts was confirmed by hemoglobin analysis and proliferation measurements. While the rate of ^{3}H-thymidine incorporation after 24 hr was constant at pH values between 7.2 and 7.9 and only slightly reduced at pH 8.1, hemoglobin expression after 72 hr was low at pH 7.2 and steadily increased with a more alkaline pH (Fig. 5B). In contrast, hemoglobin accumulation and ^{3}H-thymidine incorporation in ts v-*sea* erythroblasts were both affected to the same extent by increasingly alkaline pH. This confirms that the observed pH effects on differentiation are indeed dependent on the presence of a functional v-*erb*A oncogene and that v-*erb*A seems to arrest erythroid differentiation without concomitant effects on proliferation.

C. Switching the v-*erb*A Oncogene Off and On: v-*erb*A May Arrest Erythroid Differentiation at Immature and Intermediate Stages

The possibility of specifically inactivating v-*erb*A bioactivity, using media of alkaline pH (pH 8.1 medium) and of turning activity on again by putting cells back to acidic medium (pH 7.2 medium; Zenke *et al.,* 1988) allowed us to study whether v-*erb*A would be able to arrest further maturation of cells at any stage of differentiation, or whether it would act only during early stages as suggested for kinase oncogenes (Beug *et al.,* 1982). Two findings important for these experiments were made in pilot experiments:

1. the differentiation arrest caused by v-*erb*A at pH 7.2 was completely reversible after times between 2 and 9 d (Zenke *et al.*, 1988, and data not shown); and
2. the proliferation behavior of ts kinase-v-*erb*A erythroblasts at nonpermissive temperature and pH 7.2 (i.e., in a differentiation-arrested state) depended on the ts kinase oncogene used. Whereas v-*erb*A-ts-v-*sea* erythroblasts exhibited only a limited proliferation potential under these conditions (Schroeder *et al.*, 1990), v-*erb*A-ts-v-*erb*B erythroblasts continuously proliferated at 42°C and pH 7.2 (Fig. 6B). For this reason, results obtained on switching v-*erb*A activity off and on will be discussed separately for the two cell types.

1. v-erbA-ts v-erbB Erythroblasts

Cells from one particularly well-growing clone (ts 167 AEV clone.E3; Zenke *et al.*, 1988) were used in all these experiments. These cells grew at 37°C with a doubling time of 16 hr, whereas after differentiation induction (42°C; pH 8.1), they exhibited a doubling time of 29 hr during the first 48 hr, thereafter gradually withdrawing from cell cycle (Fig. 6A). When cultivated at 42°C and pH 7.2, the cells proliferated with a doubling time of 26 hr for more than 7 days, possibly owing to the *leakiness* of the ts mutation in v-*erb*B (Fig. 6B, and data not shown). When switched from pH 7.2 medium to pH 8.1 medium at 42°C or to normal growth medium at 37°C, cells grew with proliferation kinetics typical for the respective conditions after a 24–48 hr *lag phase* of slow growth (Fig. 6B; seen also in v-*erbA*-ts v-*sea* erythroblasts under comparable conditions; Schroeder *et al.*, 1990).

When tested for differentiation under these various conditions, ts 167-AEV E3 cells, as expected, differentated with normal kinetics at pH 8.1 whereas their maturation was completely arrested at pH 7.2 (Fig. 6C; left panels). When induced to differentiate at pH 8.1 at 42°C for 1, 2, or 3 d and then exposed to a reactivated v-*erb*A oncogene by cultivation in pH 7.2 medium, cells slowly reverted to undifferentiated cells after 1 day at pH 8.1 (Fig. 6C; upper right panel), whereas they were arrested at the state of differentiation attained after 48 and 72 hr at pH 8.1 for a further 24 to 48 hr, thereafter undergoing erythroid differentiation in a drastically slowed down fashion (Fig. 6C; middle and lower right panels). These results raise the interesting possibility that v-*erb*A might be able to arrest or at least slow down

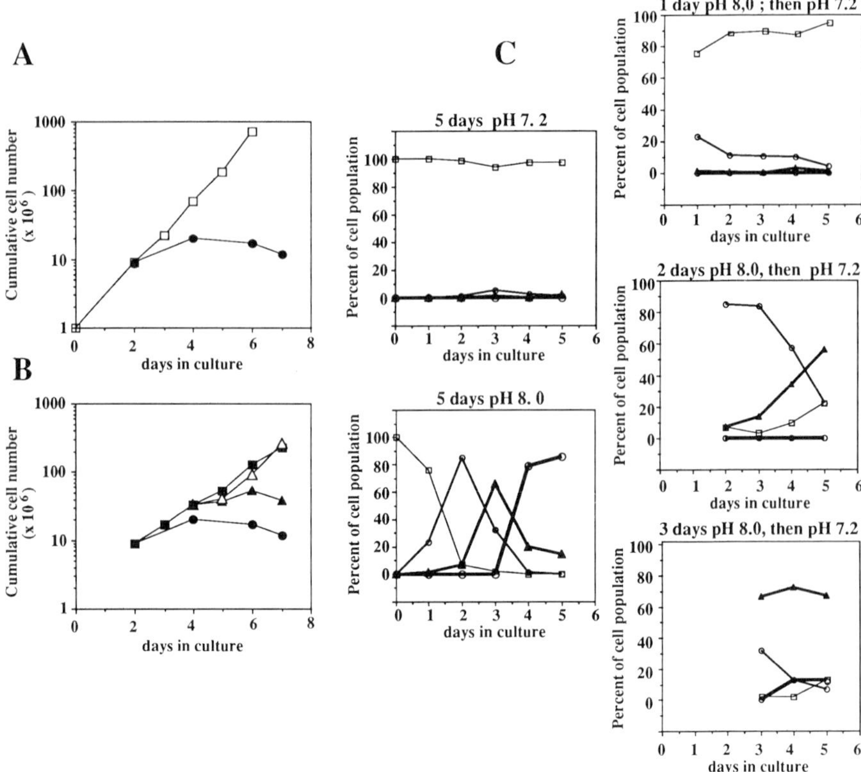

Fig. 6. Proliferation and differentiation of v-*erb*A-ts v-*erb*B erythroblasts switched between media activating or inactivating v-*erb*A. (A, B) Cells (ts 167 AEV clone E3) were cultivated at 37°C (A, open squares) or at 42°C at pH 8.1 (A,B; solid circles) or at pH 7.2 (B, solid squares). After 2 days at pH 7.2, cells were switched to pH 8.1 (B, solid triangles) or shifted back to 37°C (B, open triangles). The former cells underwent terminal differentiation, while the latter proliferated as immature erythroblasts, indicating that the cells had not been committed at pH 7.2. (C) Cells of the same clone were cultivated at 42°C and pH 7.2 or 8.0 continuously (left panels) or induced to differentiate at pH 8.0 for 1, 2, or 3 days and then switched to pH 7.2 medium (right panels). Aliquots were analyzed for differentiation by cytocentrifugation and neutral benzidine staining at the times indicated. The percentages of differentiated cell types [Ebl (squares, thin lines), ER (circles, medium lines), LR (triangles, medium to thick lines) and Ery (circles, thick lines)] were determined as described in the legend of Fig. 1.

erythroid differentiation at early, intermediate, and late stages with similar efficiency.

2. *v-erbA-ts v-sea Erythroblasts*

To investigate whether v-*erb*A was also able to arrest erythroid differentiation at different stages in v-*erb*A-ts v-*sea* erythroblasts (clone F1; Zenke *et al.*, 1988; Schroeder *et al.*, 1990), cells were induced to differentiate in pH 8.1 medium at 42°C for 24 or 48 hr and then switched back to pH 7.2 medium (Fig. 7B). Control cells were treated identically to the pH-switched cells, but reseeded into pH 8.1 medium (Fig. 7A). As expected (Kowenz *et al.*, 1987; Schroeder *et al.*, 1990), both pH 8.1 control cells and cells kept in pH 8.1 medium without manipulations (see Materials and Methods) differentiated into erythrocytes within 4 to 5 days (Fig. 7A). In contrast, cells switched back to pH 7.2 medium after 24 and 48 hr in pH 8.1 medium were efficiently arrested for 24 to 48 hr at the stage of differentiation attained after these times, and thereafter matured with grossly retarded kinetics. Surprisingly, cells underwent a sharp decline in proliferative activity after both 24 and 48 hr at pH 8.1, but thereafter retained their residual proliferation activity for at least 48 hr more (Fig. 7B). Whereas the initial drop in ^{3}H-thymidine incorporation was not unexpected (since almost any change in medium conditions leading to an altered proliferation/differentiation behavior caused a transient decrease in proliferation rate; see above and Schroeder *et al.*, 1990), the conservation of intermediate or slow proliferation rates in the partially differentiated cell populations obtained after 24- or 48-hr pH 8.1 pulses, respectively, corroborates the idea that v-*erb*A is indeed able to arrest differenting progenitors at different stages of maturation (Fig. 7B).

D. Terminal Differentiation of ts-Kinase Oncogene-Transformed Erythroid Progenitors Proceeds Normally in Absence of Cell Divisions

In myoblasts (Falcone *et al.*, 1984) and myelomonocytic cells (Beug *et al.*, 1987), terminal differentiation, although normally occuring after a fixed number of cell divisions, could also proceed in absence of a functional cell cycle, if the cells were treated with drugs inhibiting DNA synthesis before differentiation induction. These two systems,

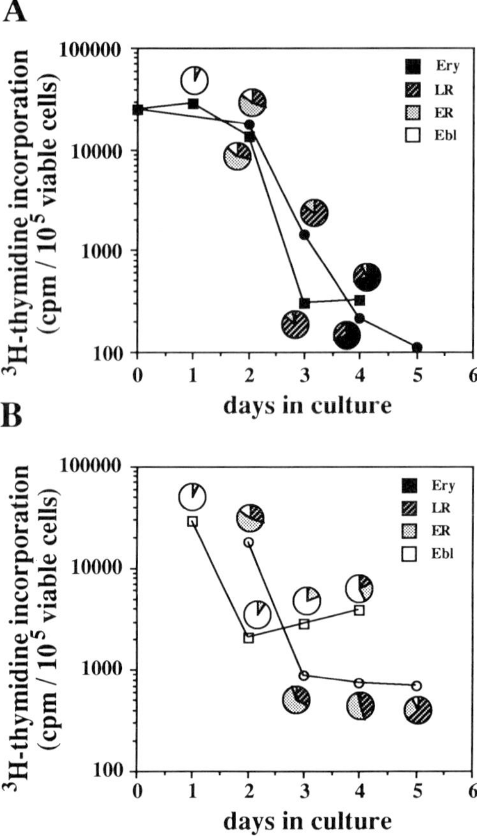

Fig. 7. Proliferation and differentiation of v-*erb*A-ts v-*sea* erythroblasts switched between media activating or inactivating v-*erb*A. (A, B) V-*erb*A-ts v-*sea* erythroblasts (clone F1; Zenke *et al.,* 1990) were induced to differentiate at 42°C in pH 8.1 medium continuously (A, solid circles). Alternatively, cells were induced in pH 8.1 medium for 24 hr (B, open squares) and 48 hr (B, open circles) and then switched back to pH 7.2 medium. As a control, cells from the same cultures as in B were mock-treated (i.e., washed and counted as for switching to pH 7.2 medium) but then reseeded in pH 8.1 medium (A, solid squares). At the times indicated, cells were analyzed for ^{3}H-thymidine incorporation and differentiation as described in the legend to Fig. 1. The states of differentiation at the different times is indicated by the pie diagrams above or below the thymidine incorporation diagrams.

however, differ from the erythroid lineage in that in myoblasts, where differentiation is irreversible as in erythrocytes, induction of muscle-specific genes commences only *after* shutdown of cell proliferation. On the other hand, differentiation of myelomonocytic progenitors, which involves cell divisions during maturation as in the erythroid system, seems to be reversible until nearly mature stages (Beug *et al.*, 1987; Ness *et al.*, 1987). It was thus of interest to determine whether erythroid progenitors that proliferate and irreversibly differentiate simultaneously during early and intermediate stages of maturation are able to differentiate with normal kinetics, if their proliferation is arrested by drugs like mitomycin C.

These studies were hampered by the problem that most drugs commonly used to arrest the proliferation of cells (e.g., hydroxyurea or aphidicolin) were toxic to differentiation-induced ts v-*sea* erythroblasts at concentrations insufficient to completely arrest cell growth. The drug mitomycin C was an exception, however, in that cells tolerated brief treatment with a dose almost sufficient to arrest proliferation (see Section IV). Accordingly, ts v-*sea* erythroblasts were treated with mitomycin C at 37°C, washed, and then induced to differentiate at 42°C in continuous presence of tritiated thymidine. Mock-treated control cells were induced to differentiate under identical conditions. After 4 d, aliquots of the cultures were cytocentrifuged onto slides and either subjected to histochemical staining for morphology and hemoglobin (Fig. 8A) or processed for autoradiography (Fig. 8B). Both mitomycin-treated and control cells differentiated into erythrocytes within this time; differentiation even seemed to be slightly more complete in the mitomycin C-treated cells (Fig. 8A). In contrast, more than 60% of the drug-treated cells failed to show any nuclear labeling, indicating that these cells had undergone terminal differentiation without a single cell division. This view is strengthened by our finding that strongly labeled cells were seen right next to unlabeled ones in the mitomycin-treated cell population (Fig. 8B) as well as by the fact that 90% of the control cells showed a strong nuclear label. Thus, the lack of nuclear label in the majority of the mitomycin-treated cells is indeed the result of an absence of cell divisions rather than due to technical problems.

III. Discussion

Conditional retroviral oncogenes (i.e., oncogene versions that can be switched on and off) have been quite useful to dissect normal and

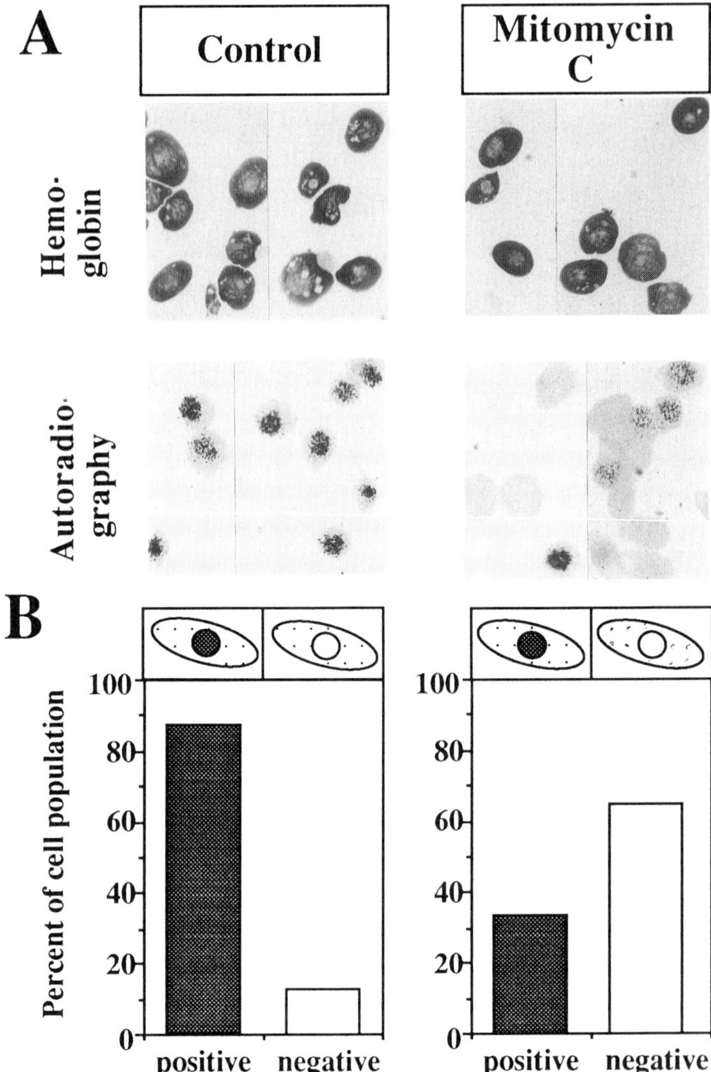

Fig. 8. Terminal differentiation of ts v-*sea* erythroblasts does not require cell division. (A) Ts v-*sea* erythroblasts (clone H2; Knight *et al.*, 1988) were treated with mitomycin (Mitomycin C) or were mock-treated with mitomycin-free medium (control) and then induced to differentiate at 42°C in presence of ^{3}H-thymidine as described in Section IV, Materials and Methods. After 4 d, aliquots from both cultures were centrifuged onto slides and either stained with neutral benzidine and photographed under blue light (hemoglobin, upper panels) or subjected to autoradiography (lower panels, see Materials and Methods) (B) Quantitative evaluation of ^{3}H-thymidine-positive (dark bars) and ^{3}H-thymidine-negative nuclei (white bars) in the cell populations shown in A .

abnormal control of proliferation and differentiation in a number of cell systems capable of differentiating *in vitro* (for review see Alema and Tato, 1987). In this chapter, we have focused on two approaches to improve the usefulness of such conditional oncogene systems. Using erythroblasts transformed by the v-*erb*A/v-*erb*B-containing leukemia virus AEV, we have tried to devise strategies to (1) switch on or off the two oncogenes independently of each other, and (2) alter the activity of one oncogene in a gradual fashion rather than just switch it on and off. By employing suitable conditional versions of c- and v-*erb*B and by modulating the bioactivity of v-*erb*A in a rather unorthodox fashion (the mechanism of which is not at all understood; Zenke *et al.,* 1988), we were indeed able to qualitatively and quantitatively control the activity of either v-*erb*B or v-*erb*A during terminal differentiation of erythroid progenitors transformed by these two oncogenes.

A. Kinase Oncogenes Abrogate Growth-Factor Dependence in and Alter the Differentiation Program of Erythroid Progenitors

In concert, the two oncogenes v-*erb*A and v-*erb*B cause proliferation of erythroid progenitors independent of hematopoietic growth factors as well as an effective arrest of erythroid differentiation at a relatively late stage (where expression of essentially all red cell proteins is already occurring; Knight *et al.,* 1988). Our trials to more clearly define the role of kinase oncogenes in this complex process using the above approach led us to several (in part tentative) conclusions. First, the onset of erythroid differentiation after turning off a kinase oncogene (by withdrawal of ligand or by raising the temperature in c-*erb*B- and v-*erb*B-transformed cells, respectively) is characterized by up-regulation of erythroid gene expression after 10 to 20 hr followed by accumulation of red cell proteins. At the same time, no significant changes in cell-cycle parameters can be detected (see Knight *et al.,* 1988). In addition, reactivation of the kinase oncogene in these cells, although rapidly arresting further accumulation of red cell proteins, caused not an increase but rather a transient decrease in proliferation rate. Finally, the speed of maturation in erythroid progenitors could be decreased progressively by expressing in them a kinase oncogene at increasing activity. The same treatment, however, did not significantly alter proliferation rate until the very late stages of differentiation

(Figs. 3, 4). This clearly suggests that c- and v-*erb*B directly alter the erythroid differentiation program rather than affecting differentiation indirectly by changing cell-cycle parameters. This view is supported by the additional finding that withdrawal of EPO during differentiation strongly slowed cell proliferation, but had only minor effects on the rates of maturation dictated by the different levels of kinase activity expressed at different temperatures (Table I; Fig. 4).

Thus, two mechanisms seem to be operative in transformation of erythroid progenitors by kinase oncogenes. First, they abrogate the dependence of erythroid progenitors to early and late erythroid growth factors (Khazaie *et al.*, 1988), and second, they partially arrest expression of many if not all erythrocyte-specific genes, leading to an (incomplete) differentiation block. Our hypothesis that this differentiation block is owing to direct effects of the kinase oncogene on erythrocyte gene transcription rather than to altered growth regulation is supported by the finding that a similar direct arrest of differentiation gene transcription is caused by kinase oncogenes in myoblasts (Falcone *et al.*, 1990). In addition, c-*erb*B/EGFR, although no longer able to abrogate EPO dependence, still induces an efficient differentiation arrest in erythroid progenitors (Khazaie *et al.*, 1988). Of course, the ligand-activated c-*erb*B oncogene probably still abrogates the requirement of erythroid progenitors for earlier growth factors (e.g. Il-3), although such factors remain to be identified in the chicken system.

It should be stressed here that immortalization, an event frequently associated with neoplastic transformation in mammalian cells (Alberts *et al.*, 1983) is not observed in any of the kinase oncogene-transformed erythroblast strains mentioned here. Although the actual *in vitro* life span of erythroblast strains is variable in different clones and also to some extent determined by the oncogene combination used (it is generally shortened in c-*erb*B erythroblast clones, but prolonged when the latter oncogene is combined with a v-*myb* oncogene; Beug *et al.*, unpublished), the ability of such clones to differentiate is not affected by the different life spans obtained in these systems. This is most obvious in the immortalized avian erythroblast line HD 3. Although growing as an immortal cell line in presence of active v-*erb*A and v-*erb*B oncogenes, the cells can readily be induced to complete terminal differentiation after turning off both oncogenes (Ullrich *et al.*, manuscript in preparation).

B. Gene Repression by v-*erb*A Can Arrest Erythroid Differentiation at Various Stages of Maturity

Our studies turning on or off v-*erb*A bioactivity in differentiating erythroblasts led us to conclude that v-*erb*A arrests or severely slows down erythroid differentiation not only at early stages but also at intermediate and late ones. At all stages, inactivation of v-*erb*A released this block and allowed terminal differentiation to proceed (Beug *et al.*, unpublished). In the presence of a weakly active v-*erb*A oncogene (i.e., at intermediate pH), differentiation proceeded in a retarded but also asynchronous fashion; that is, different cells of the same clone matured with different kinetics (Fig. 5A).

Similarly, as seen with kinase oncogenes, the rather extensive modulation of the erythroid differentiation program by v-*erb*A was not accompanied by respective changes in proliferation rate. Under all experimental conditions, cell proliferation slowed and finally ceased during late stages of erythroid differentiation (late reticulocytes to erythrocytes). However, an arrest at early stages of differentiation by v-*erb*A was both compatible with active proliferation (in presence of a temperature-inactivated v-*erb*B oncogene probably displaying a residual oncogene activity; Fig. 6A), or with an almost stationary phase characterized by doubling times of >120 hr (in presence of an inactive ts v-*sea* oncogene at 42°C, Schroeder *et al.*, 1990). Interestingly, the latter cells retained their residual ability to proliferate when arrested at intermediate stages of maturity by v-*erb*A (Fig. 7B). This observation is in line with the speculative view that the loss of proliferative potential late in erythroid differentiation is the result of certain features of erythrocytes incompatible with cell growth (i.e., degradation of organelles like ribosomes and mitochondria, as well as proteolysis of housekeeping enzymes) rather than due to a genetic program like *programmed cell death* (Alberts *et al.*, 1983).

A similar situation may well be true for myotubes. If a conditional ts v-*src* oncogene is reactivated in such terminally differentiated cells, expression of muscle-specific genes is efficiently repressed, but no division of the nuclei occurs, and DNA synthesis is not or inefficiently induced (Alema and Tato, 1987; Falcone *et al.*, 1990). It is possible that the highly specialized myotube may have lost some important components of the cell-cycle machinery and thus disintegrates rather than dedifferentiates, if expression of muscle proteins is shut down by v-*src*. The observation that differentiated cells retaining their ability to divide (e.g., fibroblasts, chondroblasts, and macrophages) can be induced to retrodifferentiate by oncogenes like v-*src* (Schwartz *et al.*, 1978; Pacifici *et al.*, 1977) or v-*myb* (Beug *et al.*, 1987) strengthens this hypothetical view.

C. Outlook

The main, slightly unorthodox conclusion suggested but not yet formally proven by the data presented in this article is that both oncogenes of the AEV virus exert their major leukemogenic effect through altering the differentiation program of erythroid progenitors. The two oncogenes strongly differ, however, in *how* they affect differentiation. While it is quite clear that v-*erb*A represses only a subset of erythrocyte-specific genes (all of which so far represent late genes), kinase oncogenes may well act on *master regulatory genes* like members of the NF-E1 family (Yamamoto *et al.*, 1990), since they reduce the expression level of most if not all erythrocyte proteins. In myotubes, ts v-*src* reexpression prevents transcription of reporter genes combined with muscle-specific promoter-enhancer combinations, but does not shut down transcription of *master* transcription factors such as myo-D or myogenin (Falcone *et al.*, 1990). One way to explain these data would be the assumption that kinases regulate the activity of transcription factors posttranscriptionally, e.g., by phosphorylation of such factors or of proteins interacting with them. Our finding that the abnormally high expression of the CA II gene in c-*erb*B/EGFR- and ts v-*sea*-transformed erythroblasts is reduced to normal, low levels a few hours after inactivating the oncogene and is as rapidly restored after reactivation of the kinase (Fig. 2; Knight *et al.*, 1988) argues that a direct action of kinase oncogenes on differentiation gene transcription might also occur in erythroblasts.

What, then, is the importance of changes in cell proliferation caused by kinase oncogenes? In discussing this question, we have to keep in mind that most *cytoplasmic* oncogenes (derived from genes involved in signal transduction) are able to abrogate the requirement for endogeneous growth factors, but (at least in avian fibroblasts) do not alter cell cycle parameters when the cells are grown in presence of such factors (Royer-Pokora *et al.*, 1978; Palmieri *et al.*, 1983). Thus, the real importance of oncogenes in growth control (at least in primary cells) seems to be their induction of autonomous, uncontrolled growth of the transformed cell, the differentiation of which has to be arrested or retarded by other mechanisms. The requirement for an oncogene effect on differentiation is particularly evident in avian myeloid cells, which can be rendered independent of myeloid growth factors by kinase oncogenes, but are not transformed by them (Fuhrmann *et al.*, 1989), most likely owing to the fact that expression of differentiation genes is not arrested but rather induced by tyrosine kinases in these cells (M. Zenke and H. Beug, unpublished).

A clear exception in this context is the v-*myc* oncogene, which drastically increases the growth rate of avian fibroblasts (Palmieri *et al.*, 1983) and is able to transform (e.g., to cause proliferation and prevent terminal differentiation in) macrophages (Graf and Beug, 1978). Interestingly, the v-*myc* oncogene seems to (partially) arrest differentiation of myoblasts into myotubes by forcing them into continuous, rapid proliferation, since these cells rapidly differentiate, if proliferation is inhibited by co-culture with normal fibroblasts (La Rocca *et al.*, 1989).

Finally, it should be stressed that the notion of oncogenes mainly altering differentiation properties of the cells they transform does not apply for immortalized tumor cells, which are the prevalent, if not exclusive type of transformed cells isolated in rodent systems. Most such immortalized cell lines clearly display an altered proliferation behavior (Alberts *et al.*, 1983). Experiments with mortal avian cell clones transformed by various conditional oncogenes and immortal lines isolated from them have made it clear, however, that transformation by oncogenes and immortalization are independent events based on different mechanisms (Ullrich *et al.*, manuscript in preparation). On the other hand, cell transformation most likely enhances the probability of a cell clone undergoing immortalization, while mutational events leading to cell transformation may occur with much higher probability if the target cell is immortalized. This interdependence of transformation and immortalization may have led to the common (but possibly wrong) idea that these two processes represent different aspects of the same basic event, that is, neoplastic transformation (Alberts *et al.*, 1983).

IV. Materials and Methods

A. Cells and Cell Culture

The origin of ts v-*sea*-transformed erythroblasts (Knight *et al.*, 1988); of v-*erb*A-ts v-*sea*- and v-*erb*A-ts v-*erb*B-erythroblasts (Zenke *et al.*, 1988); and of c-*erb*B/EGFR erythroblasts (Khazaie *et al.*, 1988) as well as the methods to culture them have been described previously. The origin of c-*erb*B/EGFR-ts v-*myb*-transformed erythroblasts will be described elsewhere (Schroeder *et al.*, manuscript in preparation). The sole reason for using these cells in some experiments was their enhanced *in vitro* lifespan at the permissive temperature, allowing generation of the required amount of cells for biochemical experiments.

B. Induction of Differentiation in Transformed Erythroblasts

In ts v-*sea* and ts v-*erb*B erythroblasts containing or lacking v-*erb*A, differentiation was induced by cultivating the cells at 42°C in differentiation medium (cells without v-*erb*A) or pH 8.1 medium (cells with v-*erb*A) containing appropriate concentrations of erythroid growth factors (EPO; Kowenz *et al.*, 1987; Zenke *et al.*, 1988). Differentiation of c-*erb*B/EGFR and EGFR-ts *myb*-erythroblasts was induced at 37°C or 42°C, respectively, by replacing EGF with EPO in the otherwise unchanged differentiation medium (Khazaie *et al.*, 1988). The medium conditions for activating or inactivating v-*erb*A function, (pH 7.2 medium and pH 8.1 medium, respectively) have been described earlier (Zenke *et al.*, 1988).

C. Modulation of ts v-*sea* Oncogene Activity at Different Temperatures

The details of this technique will be described elsewhere. Briefly, cells were induced to differentiate in specially designed, water-jacketed incubators of small size, which were heated by circulating water from accurate thermostats. The particular design of these incubators allowed maintainance of a given temperature with an accuracy of 0.05

to 0.1°C over several days, as verified by electronic thermometers connected to a recording device. Control of CO_2 and moisture was effected by adding the appropriate air–CO_2 mixtures to the incubators and keeping the culture dishes in moist chambers, respectively.

D. Modulation of v-*erb*A Bioactivity by Media of Different pH

Media with pH 7.2 to 8.2 were generated by varying the proportion of NaCl versus $NaHCO_3$ plus incubation at either 2% or 10% CO_2 as described elsewhere (Damm *et al.*, 1987). Cells were induced to differentiate in these media at 42°C as described.

E. Analysis of Erythroid Differentiation Markers

Hemoglobin content of erythroblasts preparations was measured as described (Kowenz *et al.*, 1987) using lysates of 1×10^8 cells/ml and respective lysates from peripheral red blood cells of adult chickens as control. Stages of erythroid differentiation (erythroblasts, Ebl; early reticulocytes, ER; late reticulocytes, LR; and erythrocytes, Ery) were analyzed by cytocentrifugation and staining with neutral benzidine plus histologic dyes (Beug *et al.*, 1982; Zenke *et al.*, 1988).

F. Cell-Proliferation Analysis

These assays were done as described previously (Khazaie *et al.*, 1988). Briefly, erythroblasts were seeded at 1×10^6 cells/ml into the respective media. After daily counting in a Coulter counter, cells were readjusted to approximately 0.8 to 1.5×10^6 cells/ml with fresh medium. Cumulative cell numbers were calculated, accounting for feeding with fresh medium and cell losses in counting, and plotted semilogarithmically against time in culture to allow determination of doubling times. Unless stated otherwise, ^3H-thymidine incorporation was measured by labeling 10^5 viable cells for 2 hr and harvesting in a cell harvester (Khazaie *et al.*, 1988).

G. Analysis of mRNA Expression

RNA preparation and analysis for expression of band 3, CA II, α-globin and c-*myb* mRNA by the slot-blot technique was done exactly as described in Zenke *et al.*, 1990.

H. Mitomycin-C Treatment and Autoradiography of ts v-*sea* Erythroblasts

Ts v-*sea* cells were treated for 2 hr at 37°C with 0.7 μg/ml mitomycin C (Sigma) in differentiation medium, washed three times, incubated for further 2 hr at 37°C, washed again, and then induced to differentiate at 42°C for 4 days in the continuous presence of 0.4 μC/ml ^{3}H-thymidine as described. Partial medium changes with ^{3}H-thymidine-containing differentiation medium were performed every day. From each cell preparation, several cytospins were prepared and either stained with neutral benzidine plus histological dyes or processed for autoradiography as described in Beug *et al.* (1987). Autoradiograms were developed after 4 wk of exposure.

References

Alberts, B., Bray, D., Lewis, J., Raff, M., Roberts, K., and Watson, J. D. (1983). Molecular Biology of the Cell. Garland Publishing, New York and London.

Alema, S., and Tato, F. (1987). Interaction of retroviral oncogenes with the differentiation program of myogenic cells. *Adv. Cancer Res.* **49**, 1–28.

Beug, H., and Graf, T. (1977). Isolation of clonal strains of chicken embryo fibroblasts. *Exp. Cell Res.* **107**, 417–428.

Beug, H., Palmieri, S., Freudenstein, C., Zentgraf, H., and Graf, T. (1982). Hormone-dependent terminal differentiation *in vitro* of chicken erythroleukemia cells transformed by *ts* mutants of avian erythroblastosis virus. *Cell* **28**, 907–919.

Beug, H., and Hayman, M. J. (1984). Temperature-sensitive mutants of avian erythroblastosis virus: Surface expression of the *erb*B product correlates with transformation. *Cell* **36**, 963–972.

Beug, H., Kahn, P., Döderlein, G., Hayman, M. J., and Graf, T. (1985). Characterization of hematopoietic cells transformed *in vitro* by AEV-H, an *erb*-containing avian erythroblastosis virus. *In* "Modern Trends in Human Leukaemia VI" (R. Neth, R. Gallo, M. Greaves, and K. Janka, eds.), Vol. 29, pp. 290–297. Springer Verlag, Berlin-Heidelberg.

Beug, H., Blundell, P. A., and Graf, T. (1987). Reversibility of differentiation and proliferation capacity in avian myelomonocytic cells transformed by *ts* E26 leukemia virus. *Genes Dev.* **1**, 277–286.

Damm, K., Beug, H., Graf, T., and Vennström, B. (1987). A single point mutation in *erb*A restores the erythroid transforming potential of a mutant avian erythoblastosis virus (AEV) defective in both *erb*A and *erb*B oncogenes. *EMBO J*, **6**, 375–382.

Damm, K., Thompson, C. C., and Evans, R. M. (1989). Protein encoded by v-*erb*A functions as a thyroid hormone receptor antagonist. *Nature (London)* **339**, 593–597.

Downward, J., Yarden, Y., Mayes, E., Scrace, G., Totty, N., Stockwell, P., Ullrich, A., Schlessinger, J., and Waterfield, M. D. (1984). Close similarity of epidermal growth factor receptor and v-*erb*B oncogene protein sequences. *Nature (London)* **307**, 521–527.

Falcone, G., Boettiger, D., Alema, S., and Tato, F. (1984). Role of cell division in differentiation of myoblasts infected with a temperature-sensitive mutant of Rous sarcoma virus. *EMBO J.* **3**, 1327–1331.

Falcone, G., Alema, S., and Tato, F. (1990). Transcription of muscle-specific genes is repressed by reactivation of pp60$^{v\text{-}src}$ in postmitotic quail myotubes. *EMBO J.*, in press.

Forrest, D., Munoz, A., Raynoschek, C., Vennström, B., and Beug, H. (1990). Requirement for the C-terminal domain of the v-*erb*A oncogene protein for biological function and transcriptional repression. *Oncogene* **5**, 309–316.

Fuhrmann, U., Vennstroem, B., and Beug, H. (1989). The myeloid cell-specific mutated growth factor receptor v-*fms* transforms avian erythroid but not myeloid cells. *Gen. Dev.* **3**, 2027–2082.

Gandrillon, O., Jurdic, P., Benchaibi, M., Xiao, J.-H., Ghysdael, J., and Samarut, J. (1987). Expression of the v-*erb*A oncogene in chicken embryo fibroblasts stimulates their proliferation *in vitro* and enhances tumor growth *in vivo*. *Cell* **49**, 687–697.

Graf, T., and Beug, H. (1978). Avian leukemia viruses: Interaction with ther target cells *in vivo* and *in vitro*. *BBA Rev. Cancer* **516**, 269–299.

Graf, T., and Beug, H. (1983). Role of the v-*erb*A and v*erb*B oncogenes of avian erythroblastosis virus in erythroid cell transformation. *Cell* **34**, 7–9.

Kahn, P., and Graf, T. (1986). "Oncogenes and Growth Control." Springer Verlag, Berlin.

Kahn, P., Frykberg, L., Graf, T., Vennström, B., and Beug, H. (1986). Cooperativity between v-*erb*A and v-*src*-related oncogenes in erythroid cell transformation. *In* "XII. Symposium for Comparative Research on Leukemia and Related Diseases." (F. Deinhard, ed.), pp. 41–50. Springer Verlag, Heidelberg.

Khazaie, K., Dull, T. J., Graf, T., Schlessinger, J., Ullrich, A., Beug, H., and Vennström, B. (1988). Truncation of the human EGF receptor leads to differential transforming potentials in primary avian fibroblasts and erythroblasts. *EMBO J.* **7**, 3061–3071.

Knight, J., Zenke, M., Disela, Ch., Kowenz, E., Vogt, P., Engel, D., Hayman, M. J., and Beug, H. (1988). *Ts v-sea* transformed erythroblasts: A model system to study gene expression during erythroid differentiation. *Genes Dev.* **2**, 247–258.

Kowenz, E., Leutz, A., Döderlein, G., Graf, T., and Beug, H. (1987). *Ts* oncogene-transformed erytholeukemia cells: A novel test system to purify and characterize avian erythroid growth factors. *In* "Modern Trends in Human Leukemia VII"

(R. Neth, R. Gallo, M. Greaves, and H. Kabisch, eds.), Vol. 31, pp. 199–209. Springer Verlag, Berlin.

La Rocca, S. A., Grossi, M., Falcone, G., Alema, S., and Tato, F. (1989). Interaction with normal cells suppresses the transformed phenotype of v-*myc* transformed quail muscle cells. *Cell* **58,** 123–131.

Ness, S. A., Beug, H., and Graf, T. (1987). V-*myb* dominance over v-*myc* in doubly transformed chick myelomonocytic cells. *Cell* **51,** 41–50.

Pacifici, M., Boettiger, D., Roby, K., and Holtzer, H. (1977). Transformation of chondroblasts by Rous sarcoma virus and synthesis of the sulfated proteoglycan matrix. *Cell* **11,** 891–899.

Palmieri, S., Beug, H., and Graf, T. (1982). Isolation and characterization of four new temperature-sensitive mutants of avian erythroblastosis virus (AEV). *Virology* **123,** 296–311.

Palmieri, S., Kahn, P., and Graf, T. (1983). Quail embryo fibroblasts transformed by four v-*myc*-containing virus isolates show enhanced proliferation but are non-tumorigenic. *EMBO J.* **2,** 2385–2389.

Royer-Pokora, B., Beug, H., Claviez, M., Winkhardt, H. J., Friis, R. R., and Graf, T. (1978). Transformation parameters in chicken fibroblasts transformed by AEV and MC29 avian leukemia viruses. *Cell* **13,** 751–750.

Sap, J., Munoz, A., Schmitt, J., Stunnenberg, H., and Vennström, B. (1989). Repression of transcription mediated at a thyroid hormone response element by the v-*erb*A oncogene product. *Nature (London)* **340,** 242–244.

Sap, J., Muñoz, A., Damm, K., Ghysdael, J., Leutz, A., Beug, H., and Vennström, B. (1986). The c-*erb*A protein is a high-affinity receptor for thyroid hormone. *Nature (London)* **324,** 635–640.

Schroeder, C., Raynoschek, C., Fuhrmann, U., Damm, K., Vennström, B., and Beug, H. (1990). The v-*erb*A oncogene causes repression of erythrocytespecific genes and an immature, aberrant differentiation phenotype in normal erythroid progenitors. *Oncogene,* in press.

Schwartz, R. I., Farson, D. A., Soo, W. J., and Bissel, M. (1978). Primary avian tendon cells in culture: An improved system for understanding malignant transformation. *J. Cell. Biol.* **79,** 672–679.

Yamamoto, M., Ko, L. J., Leonard, M. W., Beug, H., Orkin, S. H., and Engel, J. D. (1990). Activity and tissue-specific expression of the transcription factor NF-E1 multigene family. *Genes Dev.* **4,** 1650–1662.

Zenke, M., Kahn, P., Disela, Ch., Vennström, B., Leutz, A., Keegan, K., Hayman, M., Choi, H. R., Yew, N., Engel, J. D., and Beug, H. (1988). V-*erb*A specifically suppresses transcription of the avian erythrocyte anion transporter gene. *Cell* **52,** 107–119.

Zenke, M., Munoz, A., Sap, J., Vennström, B., and Beug, H. (1990). V-*erb*A oncogene activation entails loss of transcriptional regulatory activity in c-*erb*A. *Cell* **61,** 1035–1049.

PART II

Nuclear Tumor-Suppressor Genes

5

The p53 Gene and Gene Product

ROBIN S. QUARTIN, CATHY A. FINLAY,
AND ARNOLD J. LEVINE

Department of Molecular Biology
Lewis Thomas Laboratory
Princeton University
Princeton, New Jersey

I. Introduction

The p53 protein was first identified 11 yr ago in studies from three independent laboratories (Linzer and Levine, 1979; Lane and Crawford, 1979; DeLeo *et al.*, 1979). The p53 protein was shown to form a complex with the SV40 large tumor antigen (T antigen) in

SV40-infected and -transformed cells (Linzer and Levine, 1979; Lane and Crawford, 1979). Embryonal carcinoma cells and chemically induced transformed cell lines were shown to have elevated levels of p53 protein using antisera from animals bearing SV40-induced tumors or immunized with these tumorigenic cell lines (Linzer and Levine, 1979; DeLeo *et al.*, 1979). Based on these observations, p53 was termed a tumor antigen that interacted with a viral oncogene product, the SV40 large tumor antigen. In a wide variety of tumor-derived transformed cell lines, the levels of p53 were shown to be elevated some 5- to 100-fold above the nontransformed cell counterpart. In a cell line transformed with a temperature-senstivie SV40 T-antigen mutant, both the transformed phenotype and p53 levels were regulated in a temperature-conditional fashion (Linzer *et al.*, 1979). The level of p53 protein in these cells was shown to be regulated at the posttranslational stage; p53 protein in a transformed cell had a longer half-life than p53 protein from nontransformed cells (Oren *et al.*, 1981; Reich *et al.*, 1983). p53 Genomic and cDNA clones were first shown to immortalize cells in culture (Jenkins *et al.*, 1984) and to cooperate with an activated *ras* oncogene to transform primary rat embryo fibroblasts (Parada *et al.*, 1984; Eliyahu *et al.*, 1984). Based on this, p53 was termed an oncogene. It became clear that this was not a satisfactory explanation when it was shown that the p53 cDNA clones that immortalized cells and cooperated with the *ras* oncogene to transform cells were all mutant p53 DNA clones and that the wild-type p53 gene failed to have these biological activities (Finlay *et al.*, 1988; Eliyahu *et al.*, 1988; Hinds *et al.*, 1989a). In fact, evidence began to emerge demonstrating that the function of the wild-type p53 gene might be to negatively regulate cell growth, and that p53 could act as a tumor-suppressor gene under some circumstances (Mowat *et al.*, 1985; Finlay *et al.*, 1989; Baker *et al.*, 1990; Diller *et al.*, 1990; Mercer *et al.*, 1990; Michalovitz *et al.*, 1990). Thus, the identity and classification of the p53 gene and protein has evolved from a tumor antigen, to an oncogene, to a tumor-suppressor gene in 11 yr. The reasons for this complex change in terminology and function reflect the multifunctional role of this protein in cancer cells.

II. The p53 Gene and Gene Product

The p53 gene is localized in a 20-kilobase pair span of DNA on the p or short arm of chromosome 17 in humans (Benchimol *et al.*, 1985) and the murine chromosome 11 (Czosnek *et al.*, 1984). The gene contains eleven exons, the first of which is noncoding and is 6–10 kb away from the remaining coding sequences (Oren *et al.*, 1983; Zakut-Houri *et al.*, 1983). This gene produces a 2.5–2.2 kilobase mRNA (Reisman *et al.*, 1988; Harlow *et al.*, 1985) and a protein that migrates at 53,000 daltons in sodium dodecyl sulfate (SDS)-polyacrylamide gels. The murine, human, chicken, rat, and xenopus p53 cDNAs have been isolated and sequenced (Soussi *et al.*, 1987; Jenkins and Sturzbecher, 1988). The murine and human proteins are about 80% homologous, and the murine and xenopus proteins, about 57% homologous. Five regions of these proteins localized at amino acid residues 13–19, 111–136, 165–175, 230–252, and 264–280 (out of 390–393 amino acids total) have extensive amino acid sequence homology of 90 to 100%. All p53 proteins share a common domain structure composed of (1) a highly acidic amino-terminal region of 75 to 80 amino acids that is predicted to form an α-helical structure, followed by (2) a hydrophobic, extended proline-rich domain that spans amino acid residues 75–150, followed by (3) a nondescript linker, and (4) a highly basic carboxy-terminal region (residues 276–390 in the mouse and 319–393 in the human) containing α helical structures and helix–turn–helix motifs (Pennica *et al.*, 1984). This carboxy-terminal domain contains the three nuclear localization signals for this protein (residues 312–318, 365–370, 375–380) (Shaulsky *et al.*, 1991), a DNA-binding domain, and a set of signals important for oligomeric protein interactions (see Table I). The structure of the p53 protein has also been probed by a series of monoclonal antibodies, some of which are conformation dependent (Yewdell *et al.*, 1986). It has been possible to map the predominant epitopes for six of these monoclonal antibodies. Antibody PAb242 recognizes an epitope between amino acids 9 and 25; PAb246, at residues 88–109; PAb2C2 and PAb248, at residues 157–192; PAb240, at residues 156–335; PAb421, at residues 370–378 (Wade-Evans and Jenkins, 1985; Yewdell *et al.*, 1986; Bartek *et al.*, 1990) (see Table I). The binding of PAb246 recognizes a conformation-dependent epitope on the wild-type p53 protein and does not bind to several different mutant p53 proteins (Tan *et al.*, 1986; Clarke *et al.*, 1988; Hinds *et al.*, 1989b). Conversely, the PAb240 antibody fails to recognize the native wild-type p53 protein but will react with some mutant p53 proteins and with the denatured wild-type protein (Bartek *et al.*, 1990; Iggo *et al.*, 1990). In general, p53 mutant proteins with missense mutations that map between amino acid residues 118 and about 250 are not bound by PAb 246 and will react with

TABLE I

The p53 Protein

Amino acid residues[a]	Domain structure	Monoclonal antibody epitopes	Functional correlates
1–75	Very acidic, alpha helical	PAb242 (9–25)	Acid blob (transactivator)
75–150	Extended, proline-rich, hydrophobic	PAb(246) (88–109)	Wild-type epitope only (88–109)
150–280	Linker region	PAb2C2 and PAb248 (157–192); PAb240 (156–335)	Mutant epitope only (156–335)
280–390	Very basic, helix–turn–helix	PAb421 (370–378)	(a) 312–318—NLS-1 312-cdc-2 kinase site 365–370—NLS-2 375–380—NLS-3 (b) Oligomeric protein site (c) DNA-binding domain

[a]Missense mutations that map between residues 118 and 307 produce p53 proteins that are activated for transformation. Hot-spot mutations are localized at amino acid residues 175, 248, 273, and 281.

PAb240, indicating that a conformational change takes place in regions of the protein located outside the local environment of the mutation.

III. The Phenotype of Mutant p53 Genes

A. Biological Properties

A wide variety of missense mutations in the p53 gene localized between amino acid residues 118 and 307 have been shown to activate the p53 gene or cDNA clones for a gain of several new biological activities. The transfection of such mutant DNA clones into primary rat embryo fibroblasts (REF) in cell culture results in a 3- to 7-fold increase in the plating efficiency of these REF cells (Finlay *et al.*, 1989), and a marked increase (about 10-fold) in the ability of these REF cells to produce permanent cell lines in culture (Rovinski *et al.*, 1987; Levine *et al.*, 1989). Cotransfection of mutant p53 DNA clones with an activated *ras* oncogene, produce transformed foci that are tumorigenic in syngeneic rats (Eliyahu *et al.*, 1988; Hinds *et al.*, 1989a,b; Frey and Levine, 1989), and when mutant p53 DNA clones are introduced into a nontumorigenic permanent cell line in culture (such as Rat-1), the cells acquire an increased potential to produce tumors in nude mice (Eliyahu *et al.*, 1985). The murine or human wild-type p53 cDNA clones fail to express any of these characteristics in culture. Missense mutations are required for each of these activities, suggesting that the altered protein product has some functional role in these assays.

B. Phenotype of Mutant p53 Proteins

The mutant p53 proteins expressed in transformed cells in culture have been studied in some detail. In virtually all cases, a transformation-activating mutation results in an increased half-life of the mutant p53 protein and correspondingly increased levels of p53 protein in a transformed cell. The half-life of wild-type p53 varies between 6 and 20 min, depending on the cell type under study (Oren *et al.*, 1981; Rogel *et al.*, 1985). All of the mutant p53 proteins that are activated for transformation have extended half-lives of 1.5 to 12 hr (Oren *et al.*, 1981; Reich *et al.*, 1983). For activating mutations that are localized between amino acid residues 118 and 250, the p53 proteins commonly have an altered conformation, indicated by a failure to bind PAb246 and the acquired ability to bind PAb240 (Yewdell *et al.*, 1986; Tan *et al.*, 1986; Clarke *et al.*, 1988; Finlay *et al.*, 1988; Bartek *et al.*, 1990). These same p53 mutant proteins, with an altered conformation, are found to complex with the cellular heat-shock protein hsc70 (Pinhasi-Kimhi *et al.*, 1986; Sturzbecher *et al.*, 1987; Hinds *et al.*, 1987; Finlay *et al.*, 1988; Clarke *et al.*, 1988). The mutant p53-hsc70 oligomeric complex has been purified to homogeneity, *and* can be dissociated by the addition of adenosine triphosphate (ATP). This process requires the hydrolysis of ATP to effect the dissociation (Clarke *et al.*, 1988). The hsc70 protein has an intrinsic ATPase, and the role of this protein appears to be to catalyze the assembly of protein complexes and possibly transport such complexes to the nucleus (Rothman, 1989). It has been suggested (Levine, 1990) that the altered conformation of mutant p53 protein results in a tighter binding, with hsc70 requiring higher ATP concentrations for release of the mutant p53 protein, as compared to the wild-type protein. This results in a trapping and accumulation of mutant p53 protein in such a complex. These oligomeric protein complexes of mutant p53 and hsc70 also have been shown to contain the endogenous rat cell wild-type p53 protein (derived from the rat cell genes of REF-transformed cells) (Finlay *et al.*, 1989), as well as an additional cellular protein of 90,000 daltons (Hinds *et al.*, 1990), which copurifies with this complex. Thus, the mutant p53 protein is localized in a complex with hsc70, the rat endogenous wild-type p53 proteins, and a 90-kda protein.

Mutant p53 proteins with mutations at amino acid residues 273 or 281 transform REF cells with a lower efficiency than do proteins with mutations between residues 118 and 250 (2.5- to 6.0-fold less well) and do not form detectable protein complexes with hsc70 protein (Hinds *et al.*, 1990). It also appears that these mutant p53 proteins (mutations at 273, 281) have less dramatic conformational alterations than the other class of mutants (mutations between residues 118 and 250). To date, two classes of missense mutant p53 proteins have been recognized: (1) those mutated between amino acid residues 118 and 250 transform REF cells efficiently with an activated *ras* oncogene, have an altered conformation, bind to hsc70, and sequester the cellular wild-type p53 in a complex; and (2) proteins with mutations at amino acid residues 273 or 281 transform cells with a lower efficiency, have a less dramatic conformational change, and do not detectably bind to hsc70 (Hinds *et al.*, 1990) (Table I). Interestingly, in human colon cancer (Baker *et al.*, 1989; Nigro *et al.*, 1989), four missense mutations, at residues 175, 248, 273, and 281, represent over 50% of the missense mutants detected in these tumors. These hot-spot mutations fall into both classes of the p53 mutations observed and selected for in these tumors (Hinds *et al.*, 1990).

The available evidence indicates that missense mutant p53 proteins can contribute to cell growth in two ways: (1) as a gain of a new function mutation, and (2) as a dominant loss of wild-type function mutation. The gain of a new function is suggested by an experiment in which a mutant p53 cDNA clone was added to a cell line that did not express any detectable p53 protein (Wolf *et al.*, 1984). The addition of a mutant p53 protein enhanced the ability of these cells to make tumors in isogenic mice. The addition of mutant p53 to a cell, in the absence of any endogenous p53, adds a new growth potential to this cell line, clearly a gain-of-function mutation. On the other hand, when mutant p53 proteins are expressed in cells that contain the wild-type p53 proteins, they form an oligomeric protein complex consisting of hsc70-mutant and wild-type p53 (Finlay *et al.*, 1989). This could permit the mutant form of the protein to inactivate or poison the normal wild-type function and so would be termed a dominant loss-of-function mutation. In a p53 plus *ras* transformed cell line, these hsc70-p53 complexes are held in the cytoplasm of the cell during the G_1 phase of the cell cycle only, entering the nucleus in S phase (Martinez *et al.*, 1990). There is a growing body of evidence that the function of the wild-type p53 proteins is to act in G_1 to regulate entry into the S phase (Diller *et al.*, 1990; Mercer *et al.*, 1990; Michalovitz *et al.*, 1990; Martinez *et al.*, 1990). Furthermore, it is clear that mutant and wild-type p53 require their nuclear localization signals to function, i.e., act in the nucleus of a cell (Shaulsky *et al.*, 1991). Thus, by sequestering the wild-type p53 in a cell, in a hsc70-mutant-wild-type p53 complex in the cytoplasm during G_1, the mutant form of p53 may act in a dominant fashion to prevent the functioning of the wild-type p53 protein in a cell (Martinez *et al.*, 1990).

IV. The Phenotype of Wild-Type p53 Protein

The wild-type p53 protein appears to play a role in negatively regulating cell division in some cell types (Levine, 1990). It is likely that the p53 protein regulates the entry of cells from G_1 into the S phase. The first indication that wild-type p53 could act dominantly to suppress transformation of cells in culture came from a series of experiments demonstrating that the wild-type p53 gene, but not mutant p53 DNA clones, could inhibit the formation of transformed cell foci by oncogenes such as the adenovirus E1A plus the *ras* oncogene (Finlay *et al.*, 1989; Eliyahu *et al.*, 1989). Whereas the wild-type p53 DNA clones had little or no effect on the plating efficiency of REF cells (nontransformed cells) in culture, the expression of wild-type p53 in transformed cells inhibited colony (foci) formation (Finlay *et al.*, 1989). Similarly, the introduction of wild-type p53 into tumor or transformed cells in culture stopped their replication (Baker *et al.*, 1990; Diller *et al.*, 1990; Mercer *et al.*, 1990; Michalovitz *et al.*, 1990). These cells were shown to be blocked between the G_1 and S border of the cell cycle (Diller *et al.*, 1990; Michalovitz *et al.*, 1990;

Martinez *et al.*, 1990). The introduction of wild-type p53 DNA clones into benign colon cells in culture did not block their cell division (Baker *et al.*, 1990). Based on these studies, it has been suggested that p53 can act as a tumor-suppressor gene negatively regulating abnormal growth of cells. Just how p53 functions to do this is at present unclear.

V. p53 Genes and Gene Products in Tumors

One of the first indications that p53 could act as a tumor-suppressor gene came from the studies of Friend virus-induced murine erythroleukemias by Benchimol and his colleagues. They showed (Mowat *et al.*, 1985; Rovinski *et al.*, 1987; Munroe *et al.*, 1988) that many erythroleukemic cells in mice have undergone mutations in the p53 gene. These mutations yield missense p53 proteins that are produced at elevated levels in the tumor cells, and that possess properties similar or identical to those of the transformation-activating mutants described in the previous section. These mutant p53 proteins often have an altered conformation (PAb246 fails to bind to them), bind to a heat-shock protein, have long half-lives, and are present at elevated levels. The p53 cDNA clones derived from these tumors will immortalize REF cells in culture when transfected and expressed in these cells (Rovinski and Benchimol, 1988). Most interestingly, when these mutant p53 genes are placed into transgenic mice, the mutated p53 protein was expressed in many tissues. Progeny derived from a founder mouse expressing a mutant p53 transgene, had a 20% incidence of tumors of several tissue types (Lavigueur *et al.*, 1989). Thus, expressing mutant p53 protein in the presence of wild-type p53 proteins (the normal mouse alleles) predisposed these animals to cancer, showing the trans-dominant loss of function phenotype. The fact that only 20% of the animals developed cancer, and this always occurred later in life (after 6 m), strongly suggests that additional events (i.e., oncogene mutations or activations) are required for the formation of a tumor.

About 75% of human colon carcinomas contain missense mutations in the p53 gene (Baker *et al.*, 1989; Nigro *et al.*, 1989). These mutations are distributed between amino acid residues 118 and 307 with hot-spot mutations at residues 175, 248, 273, and 281 (Hinds *et al.*, 1990). In addition, these mutations all cluster in the most evolutionarily conserved regions of the gene at amino acid residues 111–136, 165–175, 230–252, and 264–280 (Soussi *et al.*, 1987). DNA clones coding for mutations at residues 143, 175, 273, and 281 were all shown to cooperate with the *ras* oncogene to transform REF cells (Hinds *et al.*, 1990). The human p53 proteins made by the 143 and 175 mutants had an altered conformation and bound to hsc70. The human p53 proteins made by the 273 and 281 mutants failed to bind to hsc70 (Hinds *et al.*, 1990) reflecting the two classes of p53 mutants. In 80% of the colon carcinomas, the second p53 allele has been lost, either by gene conversion or deletion, resulting in a reduction to homozygosity of the p53 mutant allele (Baker *et al.*, 1989).

A number of other human tumors have also been shown to have a reduction to homozygosity for the p53 locus as well as mutations in the p53 gene (Borgstrom *et al.*, 1982; Yokota *et al.*, 1987; Mackay *et al.*, 1988; James *et al.*, 1989; Tsai *et al.*, 1990) or chromosome rearrangements of the p53 gene (Masuda *et al.*, 1987; Kelman *et al.*, 1989; Ahuja *et al.*, 1989; Takahashi *et al.*, 1989). These tumors include breast, small-cell lung, bladder, astrocytomas, osteogenic sarcomas, and chronic myelogenous leukemias. In all cases, the reduction to homozygosity or the mutations in both p53 alleles suggest that the wild-type p53 protein is acting as a tumor-suppressor gene. The selection of hot-spot mutations and the clonal nature of these tumors (all the tumor cells have the same mutations) as well as the common presence of a p53 missense protein with a common phenotype, all suggest that p53 mutations are selected for in these cancer cells. This, in turn, indicates that p53 could play an active role in tumor progression via a dominant loss-of-function mutation diminishing the wild-type p53 growth-suppressor activity, and in the development of carcinomas in which a gain-of-function mutation drives the replication of these cells.

Clearly, not all tumors suffer mutations at the p53 locus. This could be because (1) the state of differentiation of a tumor or cell type might be critical to the role of p53 as a tumor suppressor; (2) there may be alternative mechanisms for inactivating p53 proteins; and (3) the different combinations of tumor suppressor genes inactivated and oncogenes activated by mutation can result in a cancer even if the p53 gene produces a normal or wild-type protein.

VI. p53 Protein Interacts with Viral Oncogene Products

The way in which the small DNA tumor viruses, such as SV40, the adenoviruses, and the papilloma viruses, transform cells in culture or initiate tumors in animals has been the subject of intense experimentation over the past 20 years. It has become clear that each of these viruses encodes two or three gene products required to transform cells in culture or produce tumors in animals (Levine, 1988). In most cases, these virus-encoded oncogenes are required both to initiate and maintain the transformed phenotype in culture. These viral-encoded oncogenes are SV40 large tumor antigen and small tumor antigen, the adenovirus E1A proteins, the E1B-19 kda and E1B-55 kda proteins, and the human papilloma virus types 16 and 18 E6 and E7 proteins. Some of these proteins have been shown to stimulate or inhibit transcription of viral and cellular genes (SV40 T antigen, adenovirus E1A proteins, HPV E7 protein), whereas other proteins appear to play a role in mRNA processing, transport, or stability (E1B-55 kda protein). Each of these viral oncogene products functions in part by interacting with cellular proteins that negatively regulate cell division (Table II). The E1A proteins, the N-terminal domain of the SV40 large T antigen, and the HPV E7 protein each bind to and presumably act on the retinoblastoma susceptibility gene product, Rb (Whyte *et al.,* 1988; DeCaprio *et al.,* 1988; Dyson *et al.,* 1989). Similarly, the SV40 large T antigen domain localized between amino acid residues 272 and 517 (Schmieg and Simmons, 1988), the adenovirus type 5 E1B-55 kda protein, and the HPV E6 protein each bind to p53 proteins in the cell (Linzer and Levine, 1979; Lane and Crawford, 1979; Sarnow *et al.,* 1982; Werness *et al.,* 1990). In the case of the SV40 large T antigen, two domains of this protein have been identified as critical for transformation of specific cells in culture; these have been mapped to amino acid residues 1–120 and 325–625 (Srinivasan *et al.,* 1989). These domains overlap the T-antigen binding sites for Rb (T antigen residues 104–114) and for p53 (T-antigen residues 272–517). A set of mutations in the SV40 large T antigen gene mapping at amino acid residues 580–584 yield T-antigen proteins that fail to aggregate into high-molecular-weight oligomers. Such oligomeric complexes of T antigen are required for the binding of p53 to T antigen (Peden *et al.,* 1989). These mutants fail to transform primary mouse embryo fibroblasts or REF 52 cells

TABLE II

The DNA Tumor Virus—p53 or Rb Interactions

Virus	Viral oncogene	Cellular tumor suppressor
SV40	Large T antigen	
	residues 104–114	Rb
	residues 272–517	p53
	residues critical for transformation: 66–82, 104–114, 325–625	
Adenovirus	E1A	Rb
	E1B-55 kda	p53
Human papilloma Virus 16, 18	E6	p53
	E7	Rb

in culture. These same mutants can transform (at a level 10-fold below wild-type) C3H 10T-½ cells in culture. This heterogeneity in phenotype could be owing to the possibility that different cell lines may well have different p53 mutant genes and proteins, which would then bypass the need for T antigen to bind to and inactivate p53 in that particular cell line. It is clear that primary mouse cells in culture have the wild-type p53 gene, and T-antigen mutants that fail to bind to p53 also fail to transform these cells (Peden *et al.*, 1989).

The E6 proteins of HPV 16 and 18 bind to p53, whereas the same proteins (E6) from HPV 6 or 11 serotypes fail to detectably bind to p53 (Werness *et al.*, 1990). This is interesting because HPV 16 and 18 are associated with a high risk of obtaining anogenital cancers, whereas HPV 6 or 11 are termed low-risk viruses, rarely associated with genital cancers. In this case, the biological properties of these viruses are well correlated with the abilities of the E6 protein to bind to p53 and inactivate its function.

With each of these virus groups, the binding or interaction of the viral-encoded oncogene product with p53 and Rb is selected for by virtue of the fact that the virus requires the cell to enter a growth phase to optimally replicate the virus. Stimulating the host cell into S phase results in the induction of cellular enzymes that synthesize deoxypyrimidine and deoxypurine precursors. It also triggers a series of events resulting in the phosphorylation of SV40 T antigen by the cell cycle-regulated protein kinase, cdc2 kinase, which is required for the initiation of viral DNA replication (Levine, 1989). Both SV40 and the papilloma viruses require cellular histone synthesis, linked to S phase, to package the viral DNA into virions. It is clear then that some viruses have evolved functions to antagonize the negative regulators of cell growth. When by chance such viruses leave their own replicative cycle and integrate into a cellular chromosome, the virus continues to produce its own oncogene products, which no longer act on the virus. The oncogene product drives cell division in the absence of viral replication, and a tumor cell arises that, under other circumstances, would have been killed by a virus infection. It is remarkable that the DNA tumor viruses that encode oncogene products and natural cancers that arise by mutation over a lifetime employ different mechanisms to act on the same target genes and gene products, p53 and Rb.

VII. The Functions of p53 Genes and Gene Products

The available evidence suggests that p53 is involved in regulating the cell cycle, perhaps by negatively controlling the entry into S phase by its actions in G_1. It could do this in one of two ways: (1) by interacting with a critical protein needed for DNA replication and blocking DNA synthesis and/or (2) by regulating (positively or negatively) transcription of several critical genes required for entry into the S phase of the cell cycle. The wild-type p53 protein binds to the domain of the SV40 large T antigen that contains an ATPase and helicase activity (Levine, 1989) and to a region of T antigen that interacts with the α-DNA polymerase of the cell (Gannon and Lane, 1987). The binding of p53 to T antigen blocks the ATP-dependent helicase activity, stops the initiation of SV40 DNA replication by T antigen (Braithwaite *et al.*, 1987; Sturzbecher *et al.*, 1988; Wang *et al.*, 1989), and blocks the binding of the alpha-DNA polymerase (Gannon and Lane, 1987). There is some reason to believe that p53 in a cell binds to a cellular protein with structure and properties analogous to those of T antigen. The p53 proteins from xenopus, mouse, and human sources each have retained (over evolutionary time) a binding site for SV40 T antigen, suggesting that selection for binding to a similar cellular protein has kept this site intact. Thus, it is possible that p53 regulates a cellular helicase or DNA replication complex that is important at the G_1–S border.

p53 could also regulate the transcription of cellular genes critical to passage from G_1 to S phase. The amino-terminal acidic blob region and the basic carboxy-terminal domain (helix-coil-helix) are structural motifs in p53 that are suggestive of a transactivator of transcription. Recently, p53 has been shown to bind to specific DNA sequences (Bargonetti *et al.*, 1991; Kern *et al.*, 1991). When p53 was fused to a known DNA-binding protein (Gal-4 protein) and tested for its ability to enhance transcription of a gene regulated by a Gal-4 DNA binding site, the p53 protein stimulated transcription of that gene (Raycroft *et al.*, 1990; Fields and Jang, 1990). Amino acid residues 1–72 from p53 were sufficient for this stimulatory activity, and interestingly, mutants of p53 that activate it for transformation block the transcriptional transactivation by this fusion protein (Raycroft *et al.*, 1990). Thus, it remains possible that p53 positively or negatively regulates a set of genes required for entry from G_1 to S phase in the cell cycle. The regulation of DNA replication and transcriptional activation are not mutually exclusive functions for the p53 protein.

References

Ahuja, H., Bar-Eli, M., Advani, S. H., Benchimol, S., and Cline, M. J. (1989). Alterations in the p53 gene and the clonal evolution of the blast crisis of chronic myelocytic leukemia. *Proc. Natl. Acad. Sci. U.S.A.* **86**, 6783–6787.

Baker, S. J., Fearon, E. R., Nigro, J. M., Hamilton, S. R., Preisinger, A. C., Jessup, J. M., van Tuinen, P., Ledbetter, D. H., Barker, D. F., Nakamura, Y., White, R., and Vogelstein, B. (1989). Chromosome 17 deletions and p53 gene mutations in colorectal carcinoma. *Science (DC)* **244**, 217–221.

Baker, S. J., Markowitz, S., Fearon, E. R., Wilson, J. K. U., and Vogelstein, B. (1990). Suppression of human colorectal carcinoma cell growth by wild-type p53. *Science* **249**, 912–915.

Bargonetti, J., Friedman, P. N., Kern, S. E., Vogelstein, B., and Prives, C. (1991). Wild-type but not mutant p53 immunopurified proteins bind to sequences adjacent to the SV40 origin of replication. *Cell* **65**, 1083–1091.

Bartek, J., Iggo, R., Gannon, J., and Lane, D. (1990). Genetic and immunological analysis of mutant p53 in human breast cancer cell lines. *Oncogenes* **5**, 893–899.

Benchimol, S., Lamb, P., Crawford, L. V., Sheer, D., Shours, T. B., Bruns, G. A. P., and Peacock, J. (1985). Transformation-associated p53 protein is encoded by a gene on human chromosome 17. *Somatic Cell Mol. Genet.* **11**, 505–509.

Borgstrom, G. H., Vuopio, P., and de la Chapella, A. (1982). Abnormalities of chromosome no. 17 in myeloproliferative disorders. *Cancer Genet. Cytogenet.* 5, 123–125.

Braithwaite, A. W., Sturzbecher, H.-W., Addison, C., Palmer, C., Rudge, K., and Jenkins, J. R. (1987). Mouse p53 inhibits SV40 origin-dependent DNA replication. *Nature* **329,** 458–460.

Clarke, C. F., Cheng, K., Frey, A. B., Stein, R., Hinds, P. W., and Levine, A. J. (1988). Purification of complexes of nuclear oncogene p53 with rat and *Escherichia coli* heat-shock proteins: *In vitro* dissociation of hsc70 and dnaK from murine p53 by ATP. *Mol. Cell. Biol.* **8,** 1206–1215.

Czosnek, H. H., Bienz, B., Givol, D., Zakut-Houri, R., Pravtcheva, D. D., Ruddle, H. F., and Oren, M. (1984). The gene and the pseudogene for mouse p53 cellular tumor antigen are located on different chromosomes. *Mol. Cell. Biol.* **4,** 1638–1640.

DeCaprio, J. A., Ludlow, J. W., Figge, J., Shew, J.-Y., Huang, C.-M., Lee, W.-H., Marsilio, E., Paucha, E., and Livingston, D. M. (1988). SV40 large tumor antigen forms a specific complex with the product of the retinoblastoma susceptibility gene. *Cell* **54,** 275–283.

DeLeo, A. B., Jay, G., Appella, E., Dubois, G. C., Law, L. W., and Old, L. J. (1979). Detection of a transformation-related antigen in chemically induced sarcomas and other transformed cells of the mouse. *Proc. Natl. Acad. Sci. U.S.A.* **76,** 2420–2424.

Diller, L., Kassel, J., Nelson, C. E., Gryka, M. A., Litwak, G., Gebhardt, M., Bressac, B., Ozturk, M., Baker, S. J., Vogelstein, B., and Friend, S. H. (1990). p53 Suppresses the growth of osteosarcoma cells and blocks cell cycle progression. *Mol. Cell. Biol.* **10,** 5772–5781.

Dyson, N., Howley, P. M., Munger, K., and Harlow, E. (1989). The human papillomavirus-16 E7 oncoprotein is able to bind to the retinoblastoma gene product. *Science* **243,** 934–936.

Eliyahu, D., Raz, A., Gruss, P., Givol, D., and Oren, M. (1984). Participation of p53 cellular tumor antigen in transformation of normal embryonic cells. *Nature (London)* **312,** 646–649.

Eliyahu, D., Michalovitz, D., and Oren, M. (1985). Overproduction of p53 antigen makes established cells highly tumorigenic. *Nature (London)* **316,** 158–160.

Eliyahu, D., Goldfinger, N., Pinhasi-Kimhi, O., Shaulsky, G., Akurnik, Y., Arai, N., Rotter, V., and Oren, M. (1988). Meth A fibrosarcoma cells express two transforming mutant p53 species. *Oncogene* **3,** 313–321.

Eliyahu, D., Michalovitz, D., Eliyahu, S., Pinhasi-Kimhi, O., and Oren, M. (1989). Wild-type p53 can inhibit oncogene-mediated focus formation. *Proc. Natl. Acad. Sci. U.S.A.* **86,** 8763–8767.

Fields, S., and Jang, S. K. (1990). Presence of a potent transcription-activating sequence in the p53 protein. *Science* **249,** 1046–1048.

Finlay, C. A., Hinds, P. W., Tan, T.-H., Eliyahu, D., Oren, M., and Levine, A. J. (1988). Activating mutations for transformation by p53 produce a gene product that forms an hsc70-p53 complex with an altered half-life. *Mol. Cell. Biol.* **8,** 531–539.

Finlay, C. A., Hinds, P. W., and Levine, A. J. (1989). The p53 protooncogene can act as a suppressor of transformation. *Cell* **57,** 1083–1093.

Frey, A. B., and Levine, A. J. (1989). p53-plus-*ras*-transformed rat embryo fibroblasts express tumor-specific transplantation antigen activity which is shared by independently transformed cell. *J. Virol.* **63,** 5440–5444.

Gannon, J. V., and Lane, D. P. (1987). The p53 protooncogene can act as a suppressor of transformation. *Nature (London)* **329,** 456–458.

Harlow, E., Williamson, N. M., Ralston, R., Halfman, D. M., and Adams, T. E. (1985). Molecular cloning and *in vitro* expression of a cDNA clone for human cellular tumor antigen p53. *Mol. Cell. Biol.* **5,** 1601–1610.

Hinds, P., Finlay, C., Frey, A., and Levine, A. J. (1987). Immunological evidence for the association of p53 with a heat-shock protein, hsc70, in p53 plus *ras* transformed cell lines. *Mol. Cell. Biol.* **7,** 2863–2869.

Hinds, P., Finlay, C., and Levine, A. J. (1989a). Mutation is required to activate the p53 gene for cooperation with the *ras* oncogene and transformation. *J. Virol.* **63,** 739–746.

Hinds, P. W., Finlay, C. A., and Levine, A. J. (1989b). The p53 protooncogene can suppress transformation by other oncogenes and mutations in the protooncogene can activate the gene for transformation. *In* "Common Mechanisms of Transformation by Small DNA Tumor Viruses, Chapter 7." (L. P. Villarreal, ed.), pp. 83–101. American Society for Microbiology, Washington, D.C.

Hinds, P. W., Finlay, C. A., Quartin, R. S., Baker, S. J., Fearon, E. R., Vogelstein, B., and Levine, A. J. (1990). Mutant p53 DNA clones from human colon carcinomas cooperate with *ras* in transforming primary rat cells: A comparison of the "hot spot" mutant phenotypes. *Cell Growth Differ.* **1,** 571–580.

Iggo, R., Gatter, K., Bartek, J., Lane, D., and Harris, A. L. (1990). Increased expression of mutant forms of p53 oncogene in primary lung cancer. *Lancet* **335,** 675–679.

James, C. D., Carlbom, E., Nordenskjold, M., Collins, V. P., and Cavanee, W. K. (1989). Mitotic recombination of chromosome 17 in astrocytomas. *Proc. Natl. Acad. Sci. U.S.A.* **86,** 2858–2862.

Jenkins, J. R., Rudge, K., and Currie, G. A. (1984). Cellular immortalization by a cDNA clone encoding the transformation-associated phosphoprotein p53. *Nature (London)* **312,** 651–654.

Jenkins, J. R., and Sturzbecher, H.-W. (1988). The p53 oncogenes. *In* "The Oncogene Handbook," (E. P. Reddy, A. M. Skalka, and T. Curran, eds.), pp. 403–432. Elsevier Science Publishers B. V., New York.

Kelman, Z., Prokocimer, M., Peller, S., Kahn, Y., Rechavi, G., Manor, Y., Cohen, A., and Rotter, V. (1989). Rearrangements in the p53 gene in Philadelphia chromosome-positive chronic myelogenous leukemia. *Blood* **75,** 2318–2324.

Kern, S. E., Kinzler, K. W., Bruskin, A., Jarosz, D., Friedman, P., Prives, C., and Vogelstein, B. (1991). Identification of p53 as a sequence-specific DNA-binding protein. *Science* **252,** 1708–1711.

Lane, D. P., and Crawford, L. V. (1979). T antigen is bound to a host protein in SV40-transformed cells. *Nature (London)* **278,** 261–263.

Lavigueur, A., Maltby, V., Mock, D., Rossant, J., Pawson, T., and Bernstein, A. (1989). High incidence of lung, bone, and lymphoid tumors in transgenic mice overexpressing mutant alleles of the p53 oncogene. *Mol. Cell. Biol.* **9,** 3982–3991.

Levine, A. J. (1988). Oncogenes of DNA tumor viruses. *Cancer Res.* **48,** 493–496.

Levine, A. J., Finlay, C. A., and Hinds, P. W. (1989). The p53 protooncogene and its product. *In* "Common Mechanisms of Transformation by Small DNA Tumor Viruses, Chapter 2." (L. P. Villarreal, ed.), pp. 21–37. American Society for Microbiology, Washington, D.C.

Levine, A. J. (1989). The SV40 large tumor antigen. *In* "Molecular Biology of Chromosome Function" (K. W. Adolph, ed.), pp. 71–96. Springer Verlag, New York.

Levine, A. J. (1990). The p53 protein and its interactions with the oncogene products of the small DNA tumor viruses. *Virology* **177,** 419–426.

Linzer, D. I. H., and Levine, A. J. (1979). Characterization of a 54,000 MW cellular SV40 tumor antigen present in SV40-transformed cells and uninfected embryonal carcinoma cells. *Cell* **17,** 43–52.

Linzer, D. I. H., Maltzman, W., and Levine, A. J. (1979). The SV40 A gene product is required for the production of a 54,000 MW cellular tumor antigen. *Virology* **98,** 308–318.

Mackay, J., Steel, C. M., Elder, P. A., Forrest, A. P. M., and Evans, H. J. (1988). Allele loss on short arm of chromosome 17 in breast cancers. *Lancet* **2,** 1384–1385.

Martinez, J., Georgoff, I., Martinez, J., and Levine, A. J. (1990). Cellular localization and cell-cycle regulation by a temperature-sensitive p53 protein. *Genes and Develop.* **5,** 151–159.

Masuda, H., Miller, C., Koeffler, H. P., Battifora, H., and Cline, M. J. (1987). Rearrangement of the p53 gene in human osteogenic sarcomas. *Proc. Natl. Acad. Sci. U.S.A.* **84,** 7716–7719.

Mercer, W. F., Shields, M. T., Amin, M., Suave, G. J., Appella, E., Ullrich, S. J., and Romano, J. W. (1990). Antiproliferative effects of wild-type human p53. *J. Cell. Biochem.* **14C,** 285.

Michalovitz, D., Halevy, O., and Oren, M. (1990). Conditional inhibition of transformation and of cell proliferation by a temperature-sensitive mutant of p53. *Cell* **62,** 671–680.

Mowat, M., Cheng, A., Kimura, N., Bernstein, A., and Benchimol, S. (1985). Rearrangements of the cellular p53 gene in erythroleukaemia cells transformed by Friend virus. *Nature (London)* **314,** 633–636.

Munroe, D. G., Rovinski, B., Bernstein, A., and Benchimol, S. (1988). Loss of a highly conserved domain on p53 as a result of gene deletion during Friend virus-induced erytholeukemia. *Oncogene* **2,** 621–624.

Nigro, J. M., Baker, S. J., Preisinger, A. C., Jessup, J. M., Hostetter, R., Cleary, K., Bigner, S. H., Davidson, N., Baylin, S., Devilee, P., Glover, T., Collins, F. S., Weston, A., Modali, R., Harris, C. C., and Vogelstein, B. (1989). Mutations in the p53 gene occur in diverse human tumour types. *Nature (London)* **342,** 705–708.

Oren, M., Maltzman, W., and Levine, A. J. (1981). Posttranslational regulation of the 54-K cellular tumor antigen in normal and transformed cells. *Mol. Cell. Biol.* **1,** 101–110.

Oren, M., Bienz, B., Givol, D., Rechavi, G., and Zakut, R. (1983). Analysis of recombinant DNA clones specific for the murine p53 cellular tumor antigen. *EMBO J.* **2,** 1633–1639.

Parada, L. F., Land, H., Weinberg, R. A., Wolf, D., and Rotter, V. (1984). Cooperation between gene encoding p53 tumour antigen and *ras* in cellular transformation. *Nature (London)* **312,** 649–651.

Peden, K. W. C., Srinivasan, A., Farber, J. M., and Pipas, J. M. (1989). Mutants with changes within or near a hydrophobic region of simian virus 40 large tumor antigen are defective for binding cellular protein p53. *Virology* **168,** 13–21.

Pennica, D., Goeddel, D. V., Hayflick, J. S., Reich, N. C., Anderson, C. W., and Levine, A. J. (1984). The amino acid sequence of murine p53 determined from a cDNA clone. *Virology* **134,** 477–482.

Pinhasi-Kimhi, O., Michalovitz, D., Ben-Zeev, A., and Oren, M. (1986). Specific interaction between the p53 cellular tumor antigen and major heat shock proteins. *Nature (London)* **320,** 182–185.

Raycroft, L., Wu, H., and Lozano, G. (1990). Transcriptional activation by wild-type but not transforming mutants of the p53 antioncogene. *Science* **249,** 1049–1051.

Reich, N. C., Oren, M., and Levine, A. J. (1983). Two distinct mechanisms regulate the levels of a cellular tumor antigen, p53. *Mol. and Cell. Biol.* **3,** 2143–2150.

Reisman, D., Greenberg, M., and Rotter, V. (1988). Human p53 oncogene contains one promoter upstream of exon 1 and a second, stronger promoter within intron 1. *Proc. Natl. Acad. Sci. U.S.A.* **85,** 5146–5150.

Rogel, A., Popliker, M., Webb, C. G., and Oren, M. (1985). p53 cellular tumor antigen: Analysis of mRNA levels in normal adult tissues, embryos, and tumors. *Mol. Cell. Biol.* **5,** 2851–2855.

Rothman, J. E. (1989). Polypeptide chain binding proteins: Catalysts of protein folding and related processes in cells. *Cell* **59,** 591–601.

Rovinski, B., Munroe, D., Peacock, J., Mowat, M., Bernstein, A., and Benchimol, S. (1987). Deletion of 5′-coding sequences of the cellular p53 gene in mouse erythroleukemia: A novel mechanism of oncogene regulation. *Mol. Cell. Biol.* **7,** 847–853.

Rovinski, B., and Benchimol, S. (1988). Immortalization of rat embryo fibroblasts by the cellular p53 oncogene. *Oncogene* **2,** 445–452.

Sarnow, P., Ho, Y. W., Williams, J., and Levine, A. J. (1982). Adenovirus E1b-58 kDa tumor antigen and SV40 large tumor antigen are physically associated with the same 54 kDa cellular protein in transformed cells. *Cell* **28,** 387–394.

Schmieg, F. I., and Simmons, D. T. (1988). Characterization of the *in vitro* interaction between SV40 T antigen and p53: Mapping the p53 binding site. *Virology* **164,** 132–140.

Shaulsky, G., Goldfinger, N., Tosky, M. S., Levine, A. J., and Rotter, V. (1991). Nuclear localization of wild-type and mutant p53 proteins is essential for their activities. *Oncogene,* in press.

Soussi, T., Caron de Fromental, C., Mechali, M., May, P., and Kress, M. (1987). Cloning and characterization of a cDNA from *Xenopus laevis* coding for a protein homologous to human and murine p53. *Oncogene* **1,** 71–78.

Srinivasan, A., Peden, K. W. C., and Pipas, J. M. (1989). The large tumor antigen of simian virus 40 encodes at least two distinct transforming functions. *J. Virol.* **63,** 5459–5463.

Sturzbecher, H.-W., Chumakov, P., Welch, W. J., and Jenkins, J. R. (1987). Mutant p53 proteins bind hsp72/73 cellular heat shock-related proteins in SV40-transformed monkey cells. *Oncogene* **1,** 201–211.

Sturzbecher, H.-W., Addison, C., and Jenkins, J. R. (1988). Characterization of mutant p53-hsp72/73 protein–protein complexes by transient expression in monkey COS cells. *Mol. Cell. Biol.* **8,** 3740–3747.

Takahaski, T., Nau, M. M., Chiba, I., Birrer, M. J., Rosenberg, R. K., Vinocour, M., Levitt, M., Pass, H., Gazadar, A. F., and Minna, J. D. (1989). p53: A frequent target for genetic abnormalities in lung cancer. *Science* **246,** 491–494.

Tan, T.-H., Wallis, J., and Levine, A. J. (1986). Identification of the p53 protein domain involved in the formation of the SV40 large T antigen p53 protein complex. *J. Virol.* **59,** 574–583.

Tsai, Y. C., Nichols, P. W., Hiti, A. L., Williams, Z., Skinner, D. G., and Jones, P. A. (1990). Allelic losses of chromosomes 9, 11, and 17 in human bladder cancer. *Cancer Res.* **50,** 44–47.

Wade-Evans, A., and Jenkins, J. R. (1985). Precise epitope mapping of the murine transformation-associated protein, p53. *EMBO J.* **4,** 699–706.

Wang, E. H., Friedman, P. N., and Prives, C. (1989). The murine p53 protein blocks replication of SV40 DNA *in vitro* by inhibiting the initiation functions of SV40 large T antigen. *Cell* **57,** 379–392.

Werness, B. A., Levine, A. J., and Howley, P. M. (1990). The E6 proteins encoded by human papillomavirus types 16 and 18 can complex p53 *in vitro*. *Science* **248,** 76–79.

Whyte, P., Buchkovich, K. J., Horowitz, J. M., Friend, S. H., Raybuck, M., Weinberg, R. A., and Harlow, E. (1988). Association between an oncogene and an antioncogene; the adenovirus E1a proteins bind to the retinoblastoma gene product. *Nature (London)* **334,** 124–129.

Wolf, D., Harris, N., and Rotter, V. (1984). Reconstitution of p53 expression in a nonproducer Ab-MuLV-transformed cell line by transfection of a functional p53 gene. *Cell* **38,** 119–126.

Yewdell, J., Gannon, J. V., and Lane, D. P. (1986). Monoclonal antibody analysis of p53 expression in normal and transformed cells. *J. Virol.* **59,** 444–452.

Yokota, J., Wada, M., Shimosato, Y., Terada, M., and Sugimura, T. (1987). Loss of heterozygosity on chromosomes 3, 13, and 17 in small-cell carcinoma and on chromosome 3 in adenocarcinoma of the lung. *Proc. Natl. Acad. Sci. U.S.A.* **84,** 9252–9256.

Zakut-Houri, R., Oren, M., Bienz, B., Lavie, V., Hazum, S., and Givol, D. (1983). A single gene and a pseudogene for the cellular tumor antigen p53. *Nature (London)* **306,** 594–597.

6

The p53 Gene in Human Cancer

SUZANNE J. BAKER AND BERT VOGELSTEIN
Oncology Center
Johns Hopkins University School of Medicine
Baltimore, Maryland

I. Introduction

The history of p53 research is brief but fascinating. p53 was discovered through its association with DNA tumor virus antigens in murine cells (Lane and Crawford, 1979; Linzer and Levine, 1979; DeLeo *et al.*, 1979). Subsequently, the gene encoding p53 was cloned and shown to transform rodent cells *in vitro*, either alone or in cooperation with an activated RAS gene (Eliyahu *et al.*, 1984; Parada *et al.*, 1984; Jenkins *et al.*, 1984). These transfection experiments, together with the demonstration that p53 gene expression was increased in a variety of chemically, virally, and spontaneously transformed human and rodent tumor cells (Crawford *et al.*, 1981; Benchimol *et al.*, 1982; Rotter, 1983; Thomas *et al.*, 1983; Koeffler *et al.*, 1986), all suggested that the p53 gene was an oncogene that could exert its growth-promoting effects if the normal (*wild-type*) gene were expressed at a high level.

Several convergent lines of evidence have more recently suggested a different role for p53 in neoplasia. First, it was found that in mouse erythroleukemias induced by Friend virus, the integration of the viral genome often interrupted the coding region of the p53 gene (Mowat *et al.*, 1985; Munroe *et al.*, 1988). Structural alterations of p53 genes were also seen in a human leukemia cell line and in a subset of human osteosarcomas (Wolf and Rotter, 1985; Masuda *et al.*, 1987). Although these structural changes could potentially *activate* the p53 gene by removing negative growth-regulatory components (such as occurs in several oncogenes, e.g., Downward *et al.*, 1984; Shore *et al.*, 1990), the data were also consistent with the idea that these alterations *inactivated* the gene product.

II. p53 in Human Tumors

A second kind of evidence came from the study of allelic losses in human tumors. Examination of several kinds of tumors (including those of the colon, lung, breast, brain, bladder, and ovary) showed that one copy of the short arm of chromosome 17 was frequently lost (reviewed in Cavenee, 1989). Detailed study of colorectal cancers demonstrated that over 75% of carcinomas lost regions of chromosome 17 (Vogelstein *et al.*, 1988). According to Knudson's model of suppressor-gene action, such allelic losses are thought to indicate the presence of a target-suppressor gene within the lost region (Knudson *et al.*, 1985). In such cases, it is presumed that one copy of the gene is deleted through a gross chromosomal event (mitotic recombination, abnormal chromosomal segregation, etc.), while the remaining allele is inactivated by a more localized mutation (missense or nonsense point mutation, small deletion, splice site mutation, etc.) (Hansen and Cavenee, 1987). To identify the gene that was the target of the allelic deletions, a small region of chromosome 17p that was commonly lost in different colorectal carcinomas was defined (Baker *et al.*, 1989). Twenty DNA probes detecting restriction fragment-length polymorphisms (RFLPs) on chromosome 17p were used to examine the patterns of allelic losses in colorectal tumors. DNA was obtained from 58 carcinoma specimens and compared to DNA from adjacent normal colonic mucosa. Allelic losses were scored if either of the two alleles present in the normal cells was absent in the DNA from the tumor cells. Seventy-seven percent of the tumors exhibited allelic losses of at least three markers. Studies of eight tumors that retained heterozygosity for some but not all markers on chromosome 17p allowed definition of a small common region of deletion, which extended between markers within band 17p12 to those within band 17p13.3. This localization is based on the assumption that the same 17p locus was the target of deletion in all of the tumors.

The p53 gene had been previously mapped to 17p13.1 (vanTuinen *et al.*, 1988), and thus became a candidate for the *target* of the allelic losses. No gross rearrangements or homozygous deletions of the p53 gene were observed in 82 colorectal carcinomas by Southern blot analysis or pulsed-field gel electrophoresis. Furthermore, normal size mRNA was detected in 22 colorectal tumors by Northern blot analysis (Baker *et al.*, 1989).

The absence of gross alterations in p53 gene structure and expression in most colorectal carcinomas did not exclude the presence of subtle alterations of the p53 gene in these cases. To test for such subtle alterations, a tumor was chosen that had an allelic deletion of chromosome 17p, yet expressed significant quantities of p53 mRNA. A cDNA clone originating from the remaining p53 allele was isolated and sequenced to determine whether the gene product was abnormal (Baker *et al.*, 1989). One nucleotide difference was identified in comparison with published p53 cDNA sequences. A transition from T to C had occurred within codon 143 (GTG to GCG), resulting in a change of the encoded amino acid from valine to alanine. The remaining p53 allele from the tumor of another patient was also sequenced and found to contain a point mutation at codon 175, resulting in the substitution of histidine for arginine (transition from CGC to CAC). For each tumor, the same change was found in the genomic DNA from both xenograft and primary tumor specimens, but was not present in normal tissue from the same patient. Thus, alterations present in the tumors were the result of specific point mutations not found in the germline of the patient, and provided evidence consistent with the idea that the p53 gene was the target of allelic deletion events in colorectal carcinomas.

To assess the timing and frequency of p53 gene mutations during colorectal tumorigenesis, a panel of 58 benign and malignant colorectal tumors (25 adenomas and 33 carcinomas) were examined for 17p allelic loss and p53 gene mutation (Baker *et al.*, 1990b). Allelic deletions are rarely seen before the carcinoma stage (Vogelstein *et al.*,

1988), and the presence of p53 gene mutations correlates strongly with the presence of allelic deletions. Of the one-allele tumors examined, 20 of 22 (91%) carcinomas and 4 of 6 (67%) adenomas contained p53 gene mutations. The frequency of these mutations was much lower in the two-allele tumors, however, with only 3 of 11 (27%) carcinomas and 2 of 19 (10%) adenomas containing p53 gene mutations. The positions of mutations in the two-allele tumors were similar to those found in one-allele tumors. A small number of tumors with allelic losses did not contain p53 gene mutations. There are two potential explanations for the lack of mutation in these tumors: (1) The remaining allele may have contained a point mutation that inactivated the gene, but was outside the previously defined region found to contain the great majority of p53 gene mutations in human tumors. For example, p53 splice-junction mutations have recently been observed in two lung tumors (Takahashi *et al.*, 1990), and one of these would not have been detected in the assay used. Similarly, a mutation in the regulatory region of the gene could have resulted in decreased or altered transcriptional or translational control of the gene, but would not have involved the coding region. Such a mutation would not have been detected; (2) It is possible that the p53 gene was not involved in the formation of these tumors. The loss of one copy of chromosome 17 may indicate the presence of a different tumor-suppressor gene located on the same chromosomal arm, or a *random* chromosomal loss associated with the increased aneuploidy found in tumors, possibly in connection with an abnormal mitotic event (Vogelstein *et al.*, 1989; Fearon and Vogelstein, 1990).

As noted above, 17p alleles are lost in a variety of human tumors. It was of interest to determine whether the remaining allele of p53 was mutated in these other tumor types. We have to date examined 48 tumors with allelic deletions of chromosome 17p including colon, breast, lung, brain, bladder, and neurofibrosarcoma (Baker *et al.*, 1989; Nigro *et al.*, 1989; Sidransky *et al.*, 1990; Baker *et al.*, 1990b). Thirty-five of the tumors were found to contain a single missense mutation; two tumors each contained two missense mutations; one tumor contained a single nonsense mutation; one tumor contained a frameshift mutation at codon 293; one tumor contained a small deletion encompassing codons 236–244; and no mutation was detected in eight tumors. Other research groups have examined the sequence of p53 alleles in a variety of tumors and have reached similar conclusions (Takahashi *et al.*, 1989; Menon *et al.*, 1990; Iggo *et al.*,

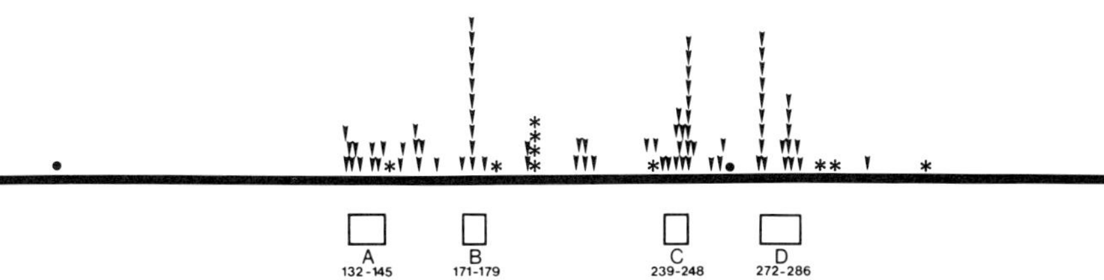

Fig. 1. p53 gene mutations cluster in four *hot-spots.* Each missense mutation is represented by an arrowhead. Nonsense mutations are denoted by an asterisk, and splice junction mutations are represented by a closed circle. The boxes below represent the four hot-spots, and comprise the codons listed below them. All human p53 gene mutations published as of October, 1990, are included in this figure (Baker *et al.*, 1989; Nigro *et al.*, 1989; Takahashi *et al.*, 1989; Menon *et al.*, 1990; Iggo *et al.*, 1990; Takahashi *et al.*, 1990; Mulligan *et al.*, 1990; Bartek *et al.*, 1990; Romano *et al.*, 1989; Cheng and Haas, 1990; Rodrigues *et al.*, 1990; Stratton *et al.*, 1990; Baker *et al.*, 1990b; Sidransky *et al.*, 1990).

1990; Takahashi *et al.*, 1990; Mulligan *et al.*, 1990; Bartek *et al.*, 1990; Romano *et al.*, 1989; Cheng and Haas, 1990; Rodrigues *et al.*, 1990; Stratton *et al.*, 1990). Taken together, these studies demonstrate that allelic deletions and concomitant point mutations of the p53 gene occur commonly in diverse human malignancies.

The vast majority of the point mutations observed were missense mutations, although nonsense, frameshift, and splice-junction alterations have also been observed. Interestingly, most mutations cluster in four hot-spots, which correspond to the four most highly conserved regions of the p53 protein (Fig. 1). Of the 41 amino acids contained within regions A–D, 93% are identical in the wild-type p53 genes of amphibian, avian, and mammalian species, compared to a conservation of only 51–57% over the entire p53 coding sequence (Soussi *et al.*, 1987; Soussi *et al.*, 1988). The clustering of mutations and evolutionary conservation of regions A–D suggest that they play a particularly important role in mediating the normal function of the p53 gene product. At the nucleotide level, the most common change was a C to T transition in the coding or non-coding strand. Presumably the spontaneous deamination of methylated cytosine residues causes CG sites to become preferential targets for mammalian point mutations (Sved and Bird, 1990). Some of the CG sites in the p53 gene have recently been shown to be methylated *in vivo* (Rideout *et al.*, 1990). An important, though speculative, conclusion from these observations is that the majority of p53 gene mutations in colorectal tumors occur as a result of cellular mistakes; there is no need to invoke carcinogenic insults to explain the pattern of mutations observed. Further discussion of this point can be found in Sommer (1990).

Allelic loss and p53 gene mutation were usually observed together in our study. It therefore could not be determined if one event consistently preceded the other. We believe, however, that point mutation precedes allelic loss in most cases. A mutation in the p53 gene probably decreases the level of functional protein through a *dominant negative* effect (Herskowitz, 1987). Oligomerization of mutant and wild-type protein may prevent the wild-type protein from interacting with other cellular factors critical for its normal function (Kraiss *et al.*, 1988). We suggest that point mutation would thereby create a stronger growth advantage for the cell than that resulting from the simple quantitative decrease in normal protein that would occur if one of two copies of the p53 gene were lost in the absence of point mutation. Once a p53 gene point mutation occurs, however, it seems that loss of the remaining allele usually follows rapidly.

III. The Role of p53 in Human Tumorigenesis

Thus, the importance of the p53 gene in human tumorigenesis is supported by a great deal of genetic evidence. Functional studies provide additional evidence that the wild-type gene may act as a suppressor of tumorigenic growth. It was observed that the p53 genes capable of transformation of rodent cells were in fact not normal, but had sustained mutations either *in vivo* or *in vitro* (Eliyahu *et al.*, 1988; Hinds *et al.*, 1989). Moreover, it was shown that wild-type murine p53 genes actually inhibited, rather than promoted, transformation of rodent cells (Finlay *et al.*, 1989, Eliyahu *et al.*, 1989).

To test the biological activity of wild-type and mutant p53 in human cells, several expression vectors were constructed for use in transfection studies (Baker *et al.*, 1990a). pCMV-Neo-Bam was engineered to contain two independent transcription units. The first unit comprised a cytomegalovirus (CMV) promoter/enhancer upstream of a site for insertion of the cDNA sequences to be expressed, and splice and polyadenylation sites to ensure appropriate processing. The second transcription unit included a herpes simplex virus (HSV) thymidine kinase promoter/enhancer upstream of the neomycin resistance gene, allowing for selection of transfected cells in geneticin. A wild-type p53 cDNA was inserted into pCMV-Neo-Bam to produce pC53-SN3. Similarly, a vector, pC53-SCX3, expressing a

TABLE I

Colony Formation after Transfection with Mutant and Wild-Type p53 Expression Vectors[a]

		Number of geneticin-resistant colonies formed	
Cell line	Experiment	pC53-SCX3 (mutant)	pC53-SN3 (wild-type)
SW837	1	754	66
	2	817	62
SW480	1	449	79
	2	364	26
RKO	1	1858	190
	2	1825	166
VACO 235	1	18	16
	2	26	28

[a]From Baker *et al.* (1990a). For each experiment, one or two 75-cm^2 flasks were transfected, and the total colonies were counted after 3 to 4 weeks of selection in geneticin (0.8 mg/ml).

mutant cDNA from a human colorectal tumor, was also constructed. The only difference between pC53-SN3 and pC53-SCX3 was a single nucleotide (C to T) resulting in a substitution of alanine for valine at p53 codon 143 in pC53-SCX3. The constructs were transfected into two colorectal carcinoma cell lines that are representative of 75% of colon carcinomas, in that each has lost one copy of chromosome 17p (including the p53 gene), and the remaining p53 allele is mutated. Geneticin-resistant colonies were counted 3 wk later. Cells transfected with pC53-SN3 formed five- to tenfold fewer colonies than those transfected with pC53-SCX3 in both recipient cell types, whereas the number of colonies produced by the expression vector pCMV-Neo-Bam (without a p53 cDNA insert) was similar to that produced by the pC53-SCX3 construct (Table I). Analysis of individual clones and pooled clones showed substantial expression of exogenous mutant sequences, whereas expression of wild-type sequences was not detectable (Fig. 2A). Results from Southern blotting were consistent with the expression studies, in that colonies from the wild-type transfectants had no detectable unrearranged exogenous p53 sequences, in contrast to the intact p53 sequences in colonies derived from the mutant p53 cDNA expression vector (Fig. 2B).

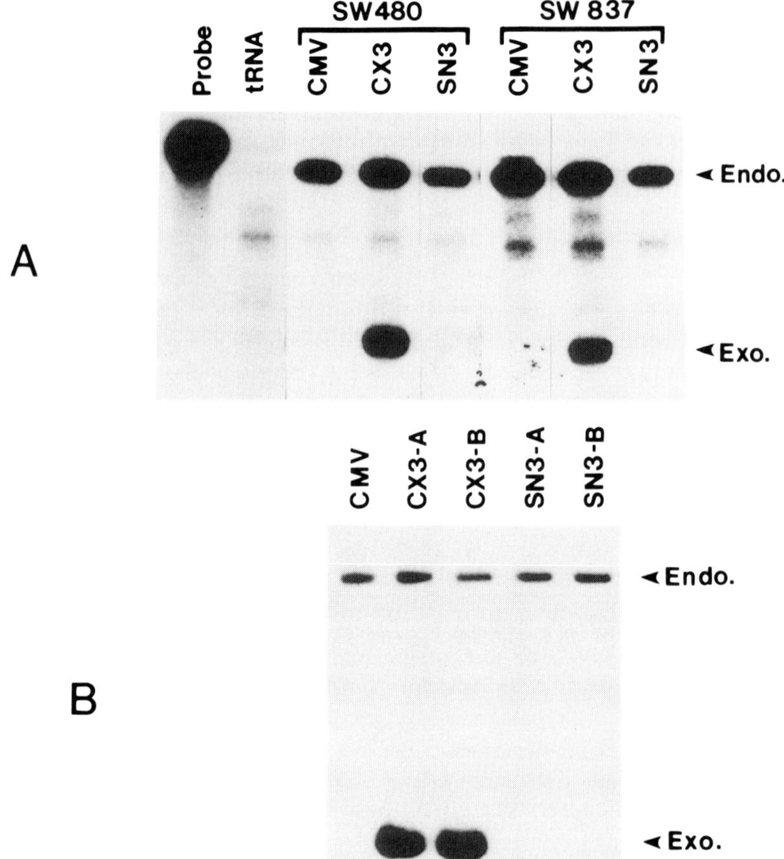

Fig. 2. (A) RNAse protection analysis of pooled clones from SW480 and SW837. A labeled probe that distinguishes between endogenous p53 mRNA and that produced from the expression vector was hybridized to total cellular RNA. Following digestion with RNAse A, the resulting hybridization products were separated on a denaturing polyacrylamide gel and autoradiographed. The endogenous mRNA produced a 388-bp hybridization product, whereas exogenous p53 message produced a 221-bp product. Lanes CMV, CX3, and SN3 contained RNA from at least 50 clones resulting from transfections with pCMV-Neo-Bam (the expression vector alone), a mutant p53 in pC53-CX3, and a wild-type p53 in pC53-SN3, respectively. Endo, endogenous; Exo, exogenous mRNA. (B) Southern blot analysis of pooled clones from SW480 cell transfectants. DNA from pooled clones was digested with *Bam*HI, separated by agarose gel electrophoresis, transferred to nylon, and hybridized to a labeled p53 gene probe. The endogenous p53 gene was present in a 7.8-kb *Bam*HI fragment (labeled Endo), and the exogenous p53 sequences gave rise to a 1.8-kb *Bam*HI fragment (labeled Exo). Lane CMV contains DNA from pooled clones following transfection with pCMV-Neo-Bam; lanes CX3-A and -B contain DNA from independent pooled clones resulting from transfection with pC53-CX3; lanes SN3-A and -B contain DNA from independent pooled clones resulting from transfection with pC53-SN3.

It was difficult to quantitatively measure protein production from the expression vectors, since these cells produced significant amounts of endogenous p53 protein that (unlike endogenous p53 mRNA) could not be distinguished from that produced by the vectors. To confirm that transfected human cells expressed p53 protein from our constructs, we studied an additional colorectal carcinoma cell line (RKO), which expressed low levels of p53 mRNA compared to those of normal colorectal mucosa or the other lines studied and did not produce detectable amounts of protein.

Immunocytochemical detection of p53 protein in transfected RKO cells revealed that approximately equal numbers of cells expressed wild-type and mutant protein 6 hr after transfection. A twofold difference was found at 24 hr, and this difference increased with time. These observations are consistent with the greater stability of mutant compared to wild-type protein noted previously (Finlay *et al.*, 1988). However, transient mRNA expression was also significantly lower in the SN3 transfectants compared to the SCX3 transfectants at 48 and 96 hr, supporting the idea that RKO cells expressing wild-type p53 were at a selective disadvantage compared to those producing mutant p53 products.

We also examined the effect of p53 gene expression on DNA synthesis in transfected RKO cells. Forty-eight hours after transfection, RKO cells were labeled with ^{3}H-thymidine for 2 hr. The cells were subsequently fixed, immunocytochemically stained for the presence of p53 protein, and autoradiographed. The number of cells undergoing DNA replication was only slightly lower in cells producing exogenous mutant p53 protein than in cells that did not express any detectable p53 protein. Expression of the wild-type protein, however, dramatically inhibited the incorporation of thymidine. A similar study in which the same expression vectors were used to transfect human osteosarcoma cells also showed that wild-type, but not mutant, p53 prevented cells from entering S phase (Diller *et al.*, 1990). Furthermore, expression of the wild-type p53 gene inhibited the growth of human glioblastoma cells (Mercer *et al.*, 1990).

These results all suggested that wild-type p53 exerted an inhibitory effect on the growth of carcinoma cells *in vitro*. To evaluate whether this inhibitory effect was cell type specific, colorectal epithelial cells derived from a benign tumor of the colon (the VACO 235 adenoma cell line) were transfected (Baker *et al.*, 1990a). Previous studies have shown that most adenomas contain two copies of chromosome 17p and express wild-type p53 mRNA at concentrations similar to that of normal colonic mucosa (Fearon *et al.*, 1987). Analogously, the p53 alleles of the VACO 235 cell line were sequenced and found to be wild type, and the expression of p53 mRNA was found to be similar to that of normal colorectal mucosa. In contrast to the results seen with the carcinoma cell lines, the wild-type and mutant expression vectors produced similar numbers of geneticin-resistant colonies after transfection of the VACO 235 line (Table I), and similar levels of exogenous p53 mRNA were transcribed from both vectors.

The combination of sequence data and transfection results suggests that cells at the premalignant stages of tumor progression (such as adenomas with two 17p alleles and no mutations, and the VACO 235 cell line) may be less sensitive to the inhibitory effects of wild-type p53 than are malignant cells. Genetic alterations that occur during the progression of colorectal tumors may increase the sensitivity of cells to p53 inhibition, making wild-type p53 expression a key, rate-limiting factor for further tumor growth and expansion. At this point, and not before, mutations in the p53 gene would confer a selective growth advantage to cells *in vivo,* which would explain the frequent occurrence of p53 gene mutations and allelic loss in only the more advanced stages of colorectal tumorigenesis. Selection for p53 point mutations and allelic deletions appears to occur at this point, and may provide an important contribution to further tumor progression.

Note (added in proof): Further evidence for the importance of the p53 gene in human neoplasia has been provided by the demonstration of germ-line mutations of p53, which predisposes patients to a variety of cancers (the Li-Fraumeni Syndrome). See Malkin, D., Li, F. P., Strong, C., Fraumeni, J. F., Nelson, C. E., Kim, D. H., Kassel, J., Gryka, M. A., Bischoff, E. Z., Tainsky, M. A., and Friend, S. H. (1990). Germ Line p53 Mutations in a familial syndrome of breast cancer, sarcomas, and other neoplasms *Science* **250,** 1233–1238; Srivastava, S., Zou, A., Pirollo, K., Blattner, W., and Cheng, C. H. (1990). Germ-line transmission of a mutated p53 gene in a cancer-prone family with Li-Fraumeni syndrome *Nature (London)* **348,** 747–749.

Acknowledgments

This work was supported through gifts from the Clayton Fund, the McAshan Fund, and grants from the U.S. National Institutes of Health.

References

Baker, S. J., Fearon, E. R., Nigro, J. M., Hamilton, S. R., Preisinger, A. C., Jessup, J. M., vanTuinen, P., Ledbetter, D. H., Barker, D. F., Nakamura, Y., White, R., and Vogelstein, B. (1989). Chromosome 17 deletions and p53 gene mutations in colorectal carcinomas. *Science* **244,** 217–221.

Baker, S. J., Markowitz, S., Fearon, E. R., Willson, J. K. V., and Vogelstein, B. (1990a). Suppression of human colorectal carcinoma cell growth by wild-type p53. *Science* **249,** 912–915.

Baker, S. J., Preisinger, A. C., Jessup, J. M., Paraskeva, C., Markowitz, S., Willson, J. K. V., Hamilton, S. R., and Vogelstein, B. (1990b). p53 gene mutations occur in combination with 17p allelic deletions as late events in colorectal tumorigenesis. *Cancer Res.,* in press.

Bartek, J., Iggo, R., Gannon, J., and Lane, D. P. (1990). Genetic and immunochemical analysis of mutant p53 in human breast cancer cell lines. *Oncogene* **5,** 893–899.

Benchimol, S., Pim, D., and Crawford, L. (1982). Radioimmunoassay of the cellular protein p53 in mouse and human cell lines. *EMBO J.* **1,** 1055–1062.

Cavenee, W., Hastie, N., and Stanbridge, E. (ed.) (1989). "Recessive Oncogenes and Tumor Suppression." Cold Spring Harbor Laboratory Press, Cold Spring Harbor, New York.

Cheng, J., and Haas, M. (1990). Frequent mutations in the p53 tumour-suppressor gene in human leukemia T-cell lines. *Mol. Cell. Biol.* **10,** 5502–5509.

Crawford, L. V., Pim, D. C., Gurney, E. G., Goodfellow, P., and Taylor-Papadimitriou, J. (1981). Detection of a common feature in several human tumor cell lines—a 53,000-dalton protein. *Proc. Natl. Acad. Sci. U.S.A.* **78,** 41–45.

DeLeo, A. B., Jay, G., Appella, E., Dubois, G. C., Law, L. W., and Old, L. J. (1979). Detection of a transformation-related antigen in chemically induced sarcomas and other transformed cells of the mouse. *Proc. Natl. Acad. Sci. U.S.A.* **76,** 2420–2424.

Diller, L., Kassel, J., Nelson, C. E., Gryka, M. A., Litwak, G., Gebhardt, M., Bressac, B., Ozturk, M., Baker, S. J., Vogelstein, B., and Friend, S. H. (1990). p53 functions as a cell-cycle control gene in osteosarcomas. *Mol. Cell. Biol.* **10,** 5772–5781.

Downward, J., Yarden, Y., Mayes, E., Scrace, G., Totty, N., Stockwell, P., Ullrich, A., Schlessinger, J., and Waterfield, M. D. (1984). Close similarity of epidermal growth factor receptor and v-*erb*B oncogene protein sequences. *Nature (London)* **307,** 521–527.

Eliyahu, D., Raz, A., Gruss, P., Givol, D., and Oren, M. (1984). Participation of p53 cellular tumour antigen in transformation of normal embryonic cells. *Nature (London)* **312,** 646–649.

Eliyahu, D., Goldfinger, N., Pinhasi-Kimhi, O., Shaulsky, G., Skurnik, Y., Arai, N., Rotter, V., and Oren, M. (1988). Meth A fibrosarcoma cells express two transforming mutant p53 species. *Oncogene* **3,** 313–321.

Eliyahu, D., Michalovitz, D., Eliyahu, S., Pinhasi-Kimhi, O., and Oren, M. (1989). Wild-type p53 can inhibit oncogene-mediated focus formation. *Proc. Natl. Acad. Sci. U.S.A.* **86,** 8763–8767.

Fearon, E. R., Hamilton, S. R., Preisinger, A. C., Willard, H. F., Michelson, A. M., Riggs, A. D., and Orkin, S. H. (1987). Clonal analysis of human colorectal tumors. *Science* **238,** 193–197.

Fearon, E. R., and Vogelstein, B. (1990). A genetic model for colorectal tumorigenesis. *Cell* **61,** 759–767.

Finlay, C. A., Hinds, P. W., Tan, T. H., Eliyahu, D., Oren, M., and Levine, A. J. (1988). Activating mutations for transformation by p53 produce a gene product that altered half-life. *Mol. Cell. Biol.* **8,** 531–539.

Finlay, C. A., Hinds, P. W., and Levine, A. J. (1989). The p53 protooncogene can act as a suppressor of transformation. *Cell* **57,** 1083–1093.

Hansen, M. F., and Cavenee, W. K. (1987). Genetics of cancer predisposition. *Cancer Res.* **47,** 5518–5527.

Herskowitz, I. (1987). Functional inactivation of genes by dominant negative mutations. *Nature (London)* **329,** 219–222.

Hinds, P., Finlay, C., and Levine, A. J. (1989). Mutation is required to activate the p53 gene for cooperation with the *ras* oncogene and transformation. *J. Virol.* **63,** 739–746.

Iggo, R., Gather, K., Bartek, J., Lane, D., and Harris, A. L. (1990). Increased expression of mutant forms of p53 oncogene in primary lung cancer. *Lancet* **335,** 675–679.

Jenkins, J. R., Rudge, K., and Currie, G. A. (1984). Cellular immortalization by a cDNA clone encoding the transformation-associated phosphoprotein p53. *Nature (London)* **312,** 651–654.

Knudson, A. G. (1985). Hereditary cancer, oncogenes, and antioncogenes. *Cancer Res.* **45,** 1437–1443.

Koeffler, H. P., Miller, C., Nicolson, M. A., Ranyard, J., and Bosselman, R. A. (1986). Increased expression of p53 protein in human leukemia cells. *Proc. Natl. Acad. Sci. U.S.A.* **83,** 4035–4039.

Kraiss, S., Quaiser, A., Oren, M., and Montenarh, M. (1988). Oligomerization of oncoprotein p53. *J. Virol.* **62,** 4737–4744.

Lane, D. P., and Crawford, L. V. (1979). T antigen is bound to a host protein in SV40-transformed cells. *Nature (London)* **278,** 261–263.

Linzer, D. I. H., and Levine, A. J. (1979). Characterization of a 54 K dalton cellular SV40 tumor antigen present in SV40-transformed cells and uninfected embryonal carcinoma cells. *Cell* **17,** 43–52.

Masuda, H., Miller, C., Koeffler, H. P., Battifora, H., and Cline, M. J. (1987). Rearrangement of the p53 gene in human osteogenic sarcomas. *Proc. Natl. Acad. Sci. U.S.A.* **84,** 7716–7719.

Menon, A. G., Anderson, K. M., Riccardi, V. M., Chung, R. Y., Whaley, J. M., Yandell, D. W., Farmer, G. E., Freiman, R. N., Lee, J. K., Li, F. P., Barker, D. F., Ledbetter, D. H., Kleider, A., Martuza, R. L., Gusella, J. F., and Seizinger, B. R. (1990). Chromosome 17 deletions and p53 gene mutations associated with the formation of malignant neurofibrosarcomas in von Recklinghausen neurofibromatosis. *Proc. Natl. Acad. Sci. U.S.A.* **87,** 5435–5439.

Mercer, W. E., Shields, M. T., Amin, M., Sauve, G., Appella, E., Romano, J. W., and Ullrich, S. J. (1990). Negative growth regulation in a glioblastoma tumor cell line that conditionally expresses human wild-type p53. *Proc. Natl. Acad. Sci. U.S.A.* **87,** 6166–6170.

Mowat, M. A., Cheng, A., Kimura, N., Bernstein, A., and Benchimol, S. (1985). Rearrangements of the cellular p53 gene in erythroleukemic cells transformed by Friend virus. *Nature (London)* **314**, 633–636.

Mulligan, L. M., Matlashewski, G. J., Scrable, H. J., and Cavenee, W. K. (1990). Mechanisms of p53 loss in human sarcomas. *Proc. Natl. Acad. Sci. U.S.A.* **87**, 5863–5867.

Munroe, D. G., Rovinski, B., Bernstein, A., and Benchimol, S. (1988). Loss of a highly conserved domain on p53 as a result of gene deletion during Friend virus-induced erythroleukemia. *Oncogene* **2**, 621–624.

Nigro, J. M., Baker, S. J., Preisinger, A. C., Jessup, J. M., Hostetter, R., Cleary, K., Bigner, S. H., Davidson, N., Baylin, S., Devilee, P., Glover, T., Collins, F. S., Weston, A., Modali, R., Harris, C. C., and Vogelstein, B. (1989). Mutations in the p53 gene occur in diverse human tumour types. *Nature (London)* **342**, 705–708.

Parada, L. F., Land, H., Weinberg, R. A., Wolf, D., and Rotter, V. (1984). Cooperation between gene encoding p53 tumour antigen and *ras* in cellular transformation. *Nature (London)* **312**, 649–651.

Rideout, W. M., Coetzee, G. A., Olumi, A. F., and Jones, P. A. (1990). 5-Methylcytosine as an endogenous mutagen in the human LDL receptor and p53 genes. *Science* **249**, 1288–1290.

Rodrigues, N. R., Rowan, A., Smith, M. E., Kerr, I. B., Bodmer, W. F., Gannon, J. V., and Lane, D. P. (1990). p53 mutations in colorectal cancer. *Proc. Natl. Acad. Sci. U.S.A.* **87**, 7555–7559.

Romano, J. W., Ehrhart, J. C., Putnu, A., Kim, C. M., Appella, E., and May, P. (1989). Identification and characterization of a p53 gene mutation in a human osteosarcoma cell line. *Oncogene* **4**, 1483–1488.

Rotter, V. (1983). p53, a transformation-related cellular-encoded protein, can be used as a biochemical marker for detection of primary mouse tumor cells. *Proc. Natl. Acad. Sci. U.S.A.* **80**, 2613–2617.

Shore, S. K., Bogart, S. L., and Reddy, E. P. (1990). Activation of murine c-*abl* protooncogene: Effect of a point mutation on oncogenic activation. *Proc. Natl. Acad. Sci. U.S.A.* **87**, 6502–6506.

Sidransky, D., Tsai, Y. C., Jones, P., Frost, P., Summerhayes, I., Von Eschenbach, A., Marshall, F., Green, P., Hamilton, S. R., Paul, M., and Vogelstein, B. (1991). The p53 gene is frequently altered in primary invasive bladder carcinoma and can be identified in urine sediment. *Science* **252**, 706–709.

Sommer, S. S. (1990). Mutagen test. *Nature (London)* **346**, 22–23.

Soussi, T., deFromentel, C. C., Mechali, M., May, P., Kress, M. (1987). Cloning and characterization of a cDNA from *Xenopus laevis* coding for a protein homologous to human and murine p53. *Oncogene* **1**, 71–78.

Soussi, T., Begue, A., Kress, M., Stehelin, D., and May, P. (1988). Nucleotide sequence of a cDNA encoding the chicken p53 nuclear oncoprotein. *Nucleic Acids Res.* **16**, 11383.

Stratton, M. R., Moss, S., Warren, W., Patterson, H., Clark, J., Fisher, C., Fletcher, C. D. M., Ball, A., Thomas, M., Gusterson, B. A., and Cooper, C. S. (1990). Mutation of the p53 gene in human soft-tissue sarcomas: Association with abnormalities of the RB1 gene. *Oncogene* **5**, 1297–1301.

Sved, J., and Bird, A. (1990). The expected equilibrium of the CpG dinucleotide in vertebrate genomes under a mutation model. *Proc. Natl. Acad. Sci. U.S.A.* **87,** 4692–4696.

Takahashi, T., Nau, M. M., Chiba, I., Birrer, J. J., Rosenberg, R. K., Vinocour, M., Levitt, M., Pass, H., Gazdar, A. F., and Minna, J. D. (1989). p53: A frequent target for genetic abnormalities in lung cancer. *Science* **246,** 491–494.

Takahashi, T., Damico, D., Chiba, I., Buchhage, D. L., and Minna, J. D. (1990). Identification of intronic point mutations as an alternative mechanism for p53 inactivation in lung cancer. *J. Clin. Invest.* **86,** 363–369.

Thomas, R., Kaplan, L., Reich, N., Lane, D. P., and Levine, A. J. (1983). Characterization of human p53 antigens employing primate-specific monoclonal antibodies. *Virology* **131,** 502–517.

vanTuinen, P., Dobyns, W. B., Rich, D. C., Summers, K. M., Robinson, T. J., Nakamura, Y., and Ledbetter, D. H. (1988). Molecular detection of microscopic and submicroscopic deletions associated with Miller-Dieker syndrome. *Am. J. Hum. Genet.* **43,** 587–596.

Vogelstein, B., Fearon, E. R., Hamilton, S. R., Kern, S. E., Preisinger, A. C., Leppert, M., Nakamura, Y., White, R., Smits, A. M. M., and Bos, J. L. (1988). Genetic alterations during colorectal tumor development. *N. Engl. J. Med.* **319,** 525–532.

Vogelstein, B., Fearon, E. R., Kern, S. E., Hamilton, S. R., Preisinger, A. C., Nakamura, Y., and White, R. (1989). Allelotype of colorectal carcinomas. *Science* **244,** 207–211.

Wolf, D., and Rotter, V. (1985). Major deletions in the gene encoding the p53 tumor antigen cause lack of p53 expression in HL-60 cells. *Proc. Natl. Acad. Sci. U.S.A.* **82,** 790–794.

7

The Retinoblastoma Protein Is Regulated by the cdc2 Kinase

QIANJIN HU, JACQUELINE LEES,
KAREN BUCHKOVICH[1], NICHOLAS DYSON,
AND ED HARLOW

Cold Spring Harbor Laboratory
Cold Spring Harbor, New York
and Massachusetts General Hospital Cancer Center
Charlestown, Massachusetts

I. Introduction

A cell's decision to divide ultimately rests on the transmission and decoding of a complicated series of signals that originate from the

[1]*Present address:* Howard Hughes Medical Institute, Department of Biochemistry, New York University Medical Center, New York, New York

environment of the cell. Extracellular molecules, which may be soluble or appropriately displayed insoluble compounds, act as cues to initiate changes in biochemical pathways. These pathways collectively pass information throughout the cell and influence the decision to initiate a cell-division cycle. Although it is known that environmental cues can provide both positive and negative signals, it is not clear whether the decision for division rests on a balance of many signals or whether it is solely a question of correctly activating a master switch.

Good experimental evidence for both positive and negative regulation of cell proliferation has been available many years, and work on the positively acting signals has been extremely successful. The transmission of negative signals is less well understood, primarily because so few members of inhibitory pathways have been identified and studied. Two avenues of experimental research have provided the major evidence for components of pathways that negatively regulate cell proliferation. First, several extracellular agents have been identified that act to inhibit cell division. Perhaps the best characterized are mating factor of yeast and TGF-β of mammalian cells (for recent reviews see Cross *et al.*, 1988; Herskowitz, 1989; Roberts and Sporn, 1990; Cross and Dexter, 1991). In both cases, when appropriate cells are treated with these agents, they arrest at specific stages of the cell cycle. The second major experimental approach has been the analysis of human tumors. During the genesis of most and perhaps all tumors, certain genes are inactivated by mutation. Here the best studied and best understood is probably the retinoblastoma gene. The loss of a functional retinoblastoma protein (pRB) is a prerequisite for tumor formation in the developing retina, presumably removing some inhibitory signal that blocks cell proliferation. The loss of pRB arises from collecting two mutations, one in each of the alleles of the retinoblastoma gene. This loss of protein function is the unifying characteristic of this class of negative regulators, now collectively known as tumor-suppressor genes. The key feature of tumor-suppressor genes is that inactivation of the gene product leads to enhanced cell proliferation or tumorigenesis. This loss is believed to remove a negative regulatory event and thus to stimulate cell proliferation (for a review of tumor-suppressor genes see Marshall, 1991).

pRB is one of the best characterized of the tumor-suppressor gene products. A number of results suggest that pRB will play a key role in regulating cell proliferation in many, if not all, cells. First, pRB is found in most cells, suggesting that pRB function is needed in most cells. Second, mutations in the RB-1 gene are found in many different tumor cells arising from various tissues. Because the loss of functional pRB is thought to be important in the development of these tumors, it is assumed that pRB is playing an important regulatory role in all of these cells. The widespread nature of the pRB protein and the selection for its loss in many different tumor types suggest strongly that the pRB function is important in many different tissues and developmental stages.

This conclusion leads to two immediate puzzles. First, if the pRB function is important to many cells, why does inheriting a mutant allele of RB-1 lead primarily to retinoblastomas and not a wide range of tumors? Children who inherit a mutation in the RB-1 gene are predisposed to develop retinoblastomas. Other tumors are seen, but normally only after the retinoblastoma has been treated. So, although the pRB mutation is found in all cells of the body, retinal cells seem to be the most sensitive to this mutation. Assuming that pRB plays has a similar function in all cells, retinal cells must be more dependent on the pRB function than other cells are. Two possibilities seem most likely to explain this dependence on pRB. Either pRB has biochemical partners that are unique to retinal cells, or retinal cells have placed more importance on the pRB regulatory pathway than other cells have. Perhaps other compensating pathways have been lost or are not relied on in retinal cells. Whatever the reason, more knowledge of the pRB biochemical pathway is needed before this puzzle can be solved.

The realization that pRB plays an important role in many cells poses a second puzzle. If pRB is present in rapidly dividing cells, how does a cell overcome its inhibitory action to allow division? Since cells do overcome the inhibitory role of pRB, its function must be regulated, and there must be a regulatory pathway that controls pRB function. Again answering this puzzle ultimately will depend on understanding the regulatory pathways in which pRB acts.

The work described here begins to address some of these questions. We have investigated the posttranslational modification of retinoblastoma protein and have found that it is phosphorylated by the cdc2 or closely related kinase. This conclusion is drawn from the observation of a physical association of pRB with cdc2, and the identification of sites on pRB that are phosphorylated *in vivo* as consensus cdc2 sites. These data suggest that pRB function is potentially regulated by the cdc2 or related kinase.

II. Results

A. Cell-Cycle Regulation of Retinoblastoma Protein

If the genetic studies correctly indicate that pRB negatively regulates cell proliferation, pRB must be controlled in some manner to allow cells to progress through the cell cycle. The regulation could occur at the level of transcription, mRNA processing, translation, or posttranslational control. However, since several groups have shown that neither the rate of pRB synthesis nor the level of pRB changes dramatically during the cell cycle (Buchkovich *et al.*, 1989; DeCaprio *et al.*, 1989; Chen *et al.*, 1989; Mihara *et al.*, 1989), it seems likely that the regulation of pRB must occur posttranslationally. Posttranslational regulation might be achieved by modification, interaction with other molecules, or changes in subcellular localization. Although none of the other regulatory mechanisms has been eliminated, the best candidate of these is modification of pRB by phosphorylation.

During the analysis of pRB throughout the cell cycle, it became clear that its relative molecular weight changed dramatically. Newly synthesized pRB is converted into slower migrating forms that, in some cells, are the only forms of the protein that can be detected on immunoblots. While these higher-molecular-weight forms can be detected by labeling cells with inorganic phosphate, the lower forms are difficult to label with phosphate. If the higher-molecular-weight forms are treated with potato acid phosphatase, they are reduced to the lower-molecular-weight forms. Together these data show that the higher-molecular-weight forms are phosphorylated derivatives of the pRB polypeptide (Buchkovich *et al.*, 1989; DeCaprio *et al.*, 1989; Chen *et al.*, 1989; Mihara *et al.*, 1989).

As might be predicted, the appearance of these phosphorylated forms of pRB is cell cycle regulated. In G_0 and G_1 phases, only unphosphorylated or underphosphorylated pRB is found. At some point before the start of S phase, highly phosphorylated forms of pRB can be detected, and these forms persist until late mitosis. This cell-cycle appearance of various forms of pRB provides a potential mechanism for disabling the negative regulatory effects of pRB. This notion is strengthened by the observations of Ludlow and colleagues (Ludlow *et al.*, 1989, 1990). They reported that SV40 large T antigen can bind only to the unphosphorylated form of pRB. Because the viral genetics of large T antigen indicated that large T antigen needs to bind to pRB to perform a required function in virus-mediated transformation, the unphosphorylated forms must encode some active function of pRB. The temporal separation of the phosphorylation of pRB during the cell cycle suggests that pRB must perform some function during the G_0 or G_1 phases of the cell cycle that can be inactivated by two alternative mechanisms; the interaction with large T, E7, or E1A would inhibit this activity, and phosphorylation would achieve similar results.

The kinases and phosphatases that regulate this transition between the phosphorylated and unphosphorylated forms then become important points of regulation for pRB. They provide one point of control and hence one level of upstream regulation. This phosphorylation event might provide one of two possible roles. It might be a master on/off switch for pRB function, enabling pRB to transmit a signal from other molecules to its appropriate targets. Alternatively, dephosphorylation at the end of mitosis might represent the only upstream signal needed to activate pRB. pRB would then carry out its biochemical activity continuously until inactivated by phosphorylation. In neither of these models is it necessary for pRB to have only one function. By the nature of our present perspective on pRB, the only functions we can analyze are those that are targeted by the viral oncoproteins. These activities appear to be restricted to the G_0 and G_1 forms.

B. cdc2 Kinase Phosphorylates Retinoblastoma Protein *in Vitro* on Sites That Are Modified *in Vivo*

We have tested several kinases in an attempt to determine which one might be capable of phosphorylating pRB. Our attention was particularly drawn to the cell cycle-regulating kinases, as their activity is well controlled during the cell cycle. To date the only kinase that we have shown to phosphorylate pRB *in vitro* is the cdc2 kinase. Purified human cdc2 can efficiently phosphorylate purified pRB. The sites on pRB that are phosphorylated *in vitro* were compared to the *in vivo* sites by two-dimensional tryptic mapping. Comparison of the authentic *in vivo* map with the *in vitro* phosphorylated pRB showed that the majority of the peptides phosphorylated *in vitro* by cdc2 are also phosphorylated *in vivo* (Lees *et al.*, 1991). This is illustrated in Fig. 1.

pRB *in vivo*

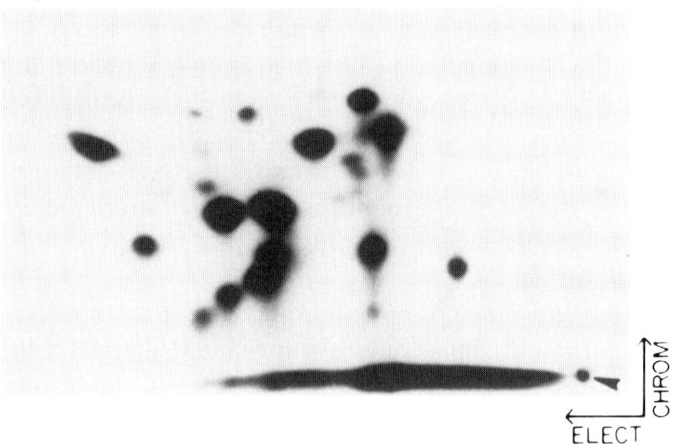

pRB *in vitro*

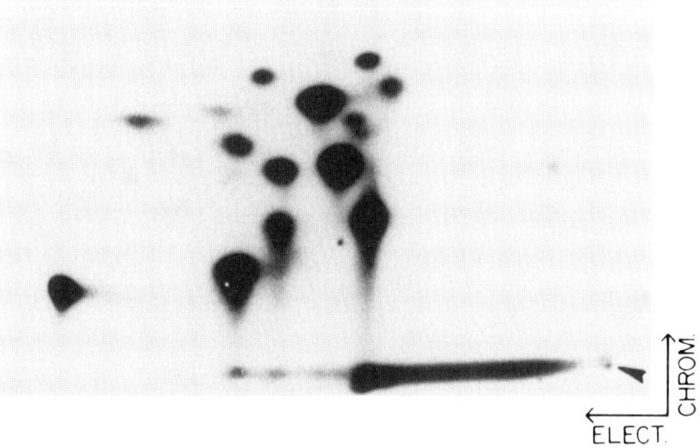

mix

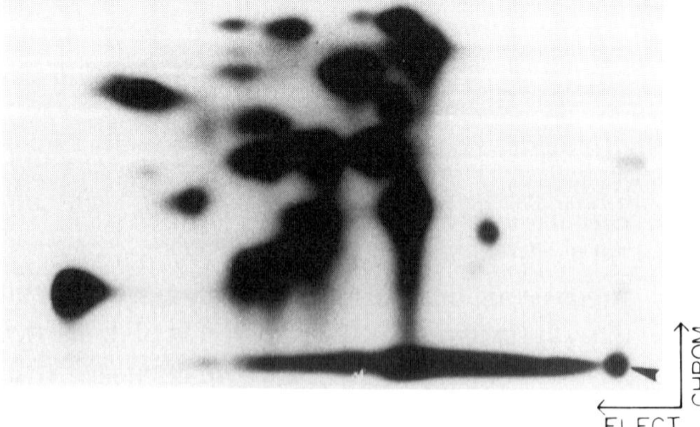

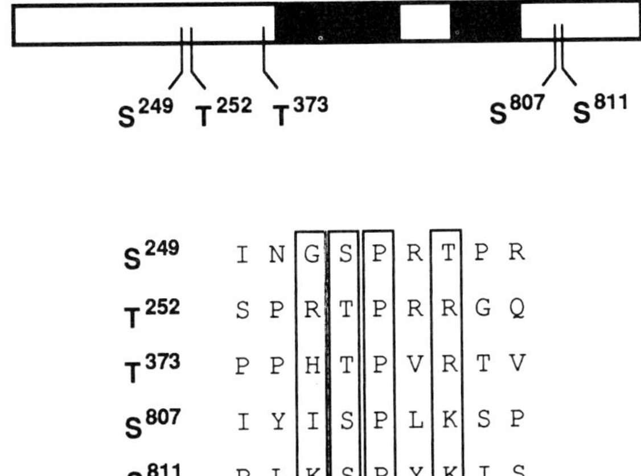

Fig. 2. Sites of phosphorylation on pRB *in vivo.* Five phosphorylation sites on pRB have been mapped to Ser-249, Thr-252, Thr-373, Ser-807, and Ser-811 (Lees *et al.,* 1991). Amino acid sequences around these sites are aligned and correspond closely to the basic/polar Ser/Thr Pro X basic consensus.

Examination of the pRB sequence reveals that it contains many sites that could potentially be substrates for the cdc2 kinase. In order to determine which sites are phosphorylated *in vivo,* we used the following strategy. Synthetic peptides that represented all of the potential cdc2 consensus phosphorylation sites were prepared and tested as substrates for the *in vitro* kinase activity of cdc2. Peptides that could be phosphorylated by cdc2 were digested with trypsin and compared with the *in vivo* phosphorylated pRB proteolytic fragments. If the peptide fragments co-migrated they were further analyzed by mass spectroscopy and amino acid sequencing (Lees *et al.,* 1991). To date, five phosphorylated residues of pRB have been identified using this strategy (Fig. 2). All of these sites contain consensus cdc2 phosphorylation sites, and therefore it appears that at least a

←

Fig. 1. Comparison of *in vivo* and *in vitro* phosphorylated pRB by two-dimensional tryptic mapping. *In vivo* phosphorylated pRB was immunoprecipitated from ML-1 cells (a human myeloid leukemia cell line) using a cocktail of anti-pRB antibodies. Unlabeled pRB was similarly prepared and incubated with purified cdc2 kinase and ^{32}P-ATP, as described in Lees *et al.* (1991). Labeled pRB was gel purified, digested with trypsin, and subjected to two-dimensional gel analysis. The top panel shows the pattern of spots generated from pRB phosphorylated *in vivo.* The middle panel shows pRB labeled by incubation with purified cdc2 kinase. The bottom panel shows a 1:1 mix of the two samples.

subset of the sites phosphorylated *in vivo* on pRB are hit by a cdc2-like kinase.

C. Retinoblastoma Protein Physically Associates with cdc2 Kinase

Given the lack of clues to pRB function, one useful approach to help determine how pRB acts is to identify proteins that physically interact with pRB. Two approaches have been used to identify such proteins. In one strategy the retinoblastoma protein itself or a fragment of it is added to cell lysates at high concentrations and used as an adsorbent for potential pRB-binding proteins. Kaelin *et al.* (1991) have used this strategy by cloning the E1A or large T antigen interaction domain of pRB as a fusion protein with glutathione *S*-transferase (GST). GST fusion proteins are bound to glutathione-agarose beads. Once bound, these beads provide a high local concentration of potential binding sites for proteins that can interact with the fusion protein. Kaelin and colleagues have identified ten proteins that can interact with a GST-pRB fusion protein (Kaelin *et al.*, 1991). In an analogous technique using high concentrations of pRB purified from overexpression in baculovirus, Wen-Hwa Lee and his colleagues (Huang *et al.*, 1991) have been able to drive pRB interactions *in vitro* and identify a 45-kDa protein that binds pRB.

We have been using a second strategy to identify interacting proteins. Using a cell line that produces high levels of pRB, we have used a new panel of monoclonal antibodies (Hu *et al.*, 1991a) to look for enzyme activities that are associated with pRB. Previously we have used these antibodies to assay for proteins that can be detected by metabolic labeling and have failed to find any proteins that we could convincingly demonstrate were bound to pRB. The analysis of associated enzyme activities allows a more sensitive test for weaker interactions. A number of the new monoclonal antibodies were able to precipitate a kinase activity that associates with pRB (Hu *et al.*, 1991b). This is illustrated in Fig. 3. Careful study of this kinase indicated that it was precipitated through its association with pRB. The same kinase was also able to phosphorylate histone H1 as an exogenously added substrate (Fig. 3). Since histone H1 is a good substrate for the cdc2 kinases, we checked to see if the associated kinase might be cdc2. Antibodies to the carboxyl-terminus of human cdc2 were able to precipitate a kinase activity that phosphorylated

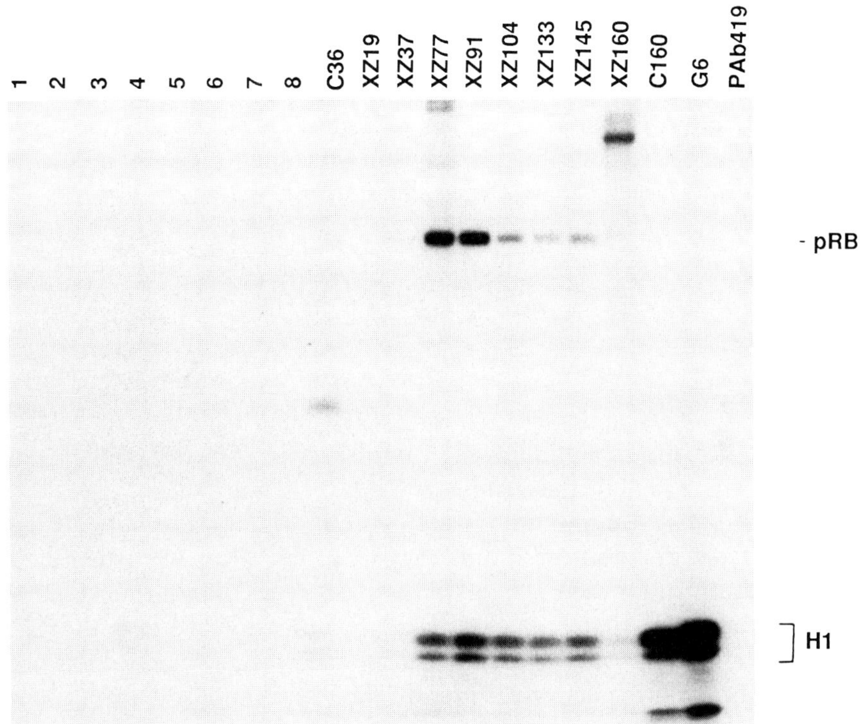

Fig. 3. pRB immunoprecipitations contain an associated kinase activity. Unlabeled ML-1 cells were immunoprecipitated with the monoclonal antibodies indicated. Lanes 1–8 contain immunoprecipitations with eight anti-pRB monoclonal antibodies purchased from Pharmigen (Rb-01–Rb-08). C36 (Whyte *et al.,* 1988) and the XZ series (Hu *et al.,* 1991a) are monoclonal antibodies to pRB. C160 is a monoclonal antibody that recognizes human cyclin A. G6 is a rabbit antisera to a carboxyl-terminal peptide from the human cdc2 sequence (Draetta and Beach, 1988). PAb416 is a negative control antibody. Immune complexes were incubated with ^{32}P-ATP in the presence of histone H1 as an exogenous substrate as described in Hu *et al.* (1991b). The entire reaction mixture was loaded onto a 6% polyacrylamide gel, and labeled proteins were detected by autoradiography. The positions of labeled pRB and histone H1 are indicated.

pRB within the immune complex. This assay revealed the presence of pRB in cdc2 immunoprecipitations. Similarly, when immune complexes containing kinase activity, which were prepared using anti-pRB antibodies, were checked for the presence of cdc2 by immunoblots, it was shown that between 1 and 5% of the total cdc2 in a cell was bound to pRB. Thus, a small fraction of cdc2 appears to be physically associated with pRB in lysates of cells.

In all these experiments cdc2 is identified using antipeptide antibodies specific for the carboxyl-terminal sequence of human cdc2 (Draetta and Beach, 1988). These data strongly suggest that cdc2 is the kinase. However, this does not preclude the possibility that the kinase is an as yet unidentified protein that is sufficiently similar to cdc2 to be recognized by antibody cross-reaction.

III. Discussion

To date, six good candidates for tumor-suppressor genes have been cloned. These include the retinoblastoma, p53, Wilm's tumor (WT-1), deleted in colon carcinoma (DCC), neurofibromatosis type 1 (NF-1), and mutated in colon carcinoma (MCC) genes. Most were identified originally through their loss in tumors. Some of these proteins have motifs that immediately suggest potential functions; others do not. Although many properties of these genes and their gene products are known, no unifying activity is found. The Wilm's tumor gene product appears to be a tissue- and stage-specific transcription factor (Call *et al.*, 1990; Rose *et al.*, 1990; Rauscher *et al.*, 1991). The DCC protein is a member of the N-CAM family of adhesion molecules (Fearon *et al.*, 1990). The NF-1 gene encodes a guanosine triphosphate (GTP)-activating protein (Buchberg *et al.*, 1990; Cawthon *et al.*, 1990; Wallace *et al.*, 1990; Xu *et al.*, 1990), whereas the MCC gene products has the motifs of a G protein (Kinzler *et al.*, 1991). The subcellular locations of these proteins differ, as do their tissue distribution. So, while the cloning of these genes has broadened our concepts of where and when negative regulation could occur, we have not learned what precepts govern negative regulation.

Two general roles can be envisioned for any factor that acts to inhibit cell growth. Negative regulators could be local governors that act on particular steps in a positive signal-transduction pathway, or they could have entire pathways of their own. Our lack of knowledge on this distinction comes from the lack of partners for negative reg-

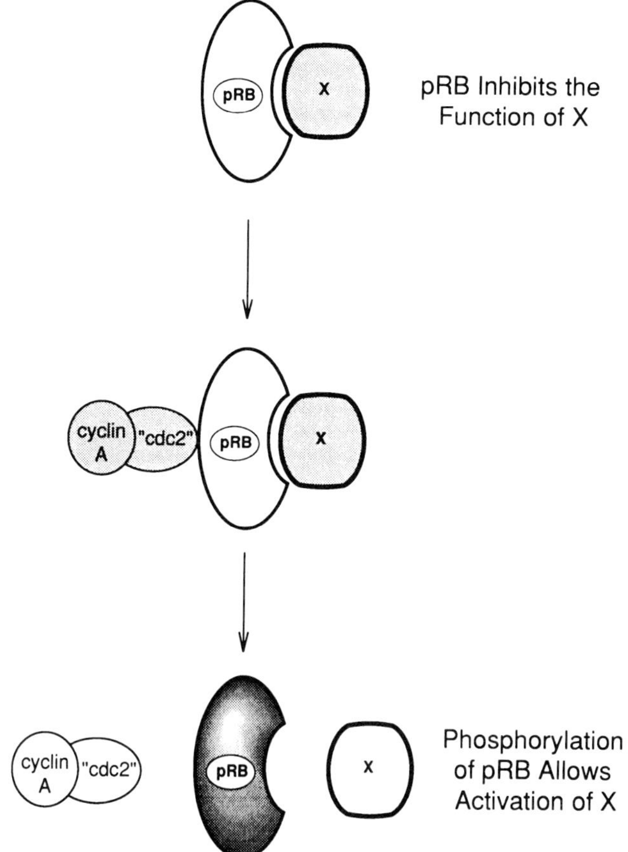

Fig. 4. Model for regulation of pRB function by cdc2 kinase.

ulators. In most cases we know little about the upstream players that control the negative regulators themselves or about the downstream targets of their action. There are many approaches to attack these questions, but one useful starting point is to identify molecules that interact with these proteins and study their role. We have examined the retinoblastoma protein and have found that it is regulated by the cdc2 kinase, one of the key proteins that control the cell cycle. This conclusion is based on the temporal pattern of pRB phosphorylation, the physical association of pRB with cdc2, and the identification of phosphorylated sites on pRB as consensus cdc2 sites. These observations suggest that the mechanisms through which pRB acts to regulate proliferation are themselves controlled by the activity of cdc2 or a closely related kinase. Current knowledge of pRB interaction with

SV40 T antigen suggests a simple model for this regulation, as illustrated in Fig. 4. In G_0 or G_1 cells, pRB inhibits the activity of an unidentified target (X). Phosphorylation of pRB by cdc2 (or a cdc2-like kinase) destabilizes the pRB/X protein complex. Dissociation of the complex releases X from pRB and allows the now-active protein to exert its positive effect on cell-cycle progression. While this model fits with our present knowledge of pRB function, other models are also possible. Attempts at model building serve merely to highlight the limits of our understanding. Clearly, the next challenge is to move from a single step in a signal-transduction pathway to the upstream and downstream partners. What is X? How is the pRB-kinase activated, and what stimulates it to phosphorylate pRB?

Acknowledgments

The experiments in the original papers were carried out in collaboration with G. Binns, D. Marshak, C. Anderson, C. Bautista, G. M. Edwards, D. Defeo-Jones and R. E. Jones. We thank L. Brizuela, J. Bischoff, K. Galactinonov, and D. Beach for generous gifts of reagents. This work was made possible by the excellent technical assistance of C. McCall and M. Falkowski. We thank colleagues at Cold Spring Harbor Laboratory and Massachusetts General Hospital Cancer Center for advice and helpful discussions. The work was supported by NIH Grant CA13106.

References

Buchberg, A. M., Cleveland, L. S., Jenkins, N. A., and Copeland, N. G. (1990). Sequence homology shared by neurofibromatosis type-1 gene and *IRA-1* and *IRA-2* negative regulators of the *RAS* cyclic AMP pathway. *Nature (London)* 347, 291–294.

Buchkovich, K., Duffy, L. A., and Harlow, E. (1989). The retinoblastoma protein is phosphorylated during specific phases of the cell cycle. *Cell* 58, 1097–1105.

Call, K. M., Glaser, T., Ito, C. Y., Buckler, A. J., Pelletier, J., Haber, D. A., Rose, E. A., Kral, A., Yeger, H., Lewis, W. H., Jones, C., and Housman, D. E. (1990). Isolation and characterization of a zinc-finger polypeptide gene at the human chromosome 11 Wilms' tumor locus. *Cell* 60, 509–520.

Cawthon, R. M., Weiss, R., Xu, G., Viskochil, D., Culver, M., Stevens, J., Robertson, M., Dunn, D., Gesteland, R., O'Connell, P., and White, R. (1990). A major segment of the neurofibromatosis type 1 gene: cDNA sequence, genomic structure, and point mutations. *Cell* 62, 192–201.

Chen, P.-L., Scully, P., Shew, Y.-J., Wang, J. Y. J., and Lee, W.-H. (1989). Phosphorylation of the retinoblastoma gene product is modulated during the cell cycle and cellular differentiation. *Cell* 58, 1193–1198.

Cross, F., Hartwell, L. H., Jackson, C., and Konopka, J. B. (1988). Conjugation in *Saccharomyces cerevisiae. Annu. Rev. Cell Biol.* **4,** 429–453.

Cross, M., and Dexter, T. M. (1991). Growth factors in development, transformation, and tumorigenesis. *Cell* **64,** 271–280.

DeCaprio, J. A., Ludlow, J. W., Lynch, D., Furukawa, Y., Griffin, J., Piwnica-Worms, H., Huang, C.-M., and Livingston, D. M. (1989). The product of the retinoblastoma susceptibility gene has properties of a cell-cycle regulatory element. *Cell* **58,** 1198–1095.

Draetta, G., and Beach, D. (1988). Activation of *cdc2* protein kinase during mitosis in human cells: Cell-cycle dependent phosphorylation and subunit rearrangement. *Cell* **54,** 17–26.

Fearon, E. R., Cho, K. R., Nigro, J. M., Kern, S. E., Simons, J. W., Rupert, J. M., Hamilton, S. R., Preisinger, A. C., Thomas, G., Kinzler, K. W., and Vogelstein, B. (1990). Identification of a chromosome 18q gene that is altered in colorectal cancers. *Science* **247,** 49–56.

Giordano, A., Whyte, P., Harlow, E., Franza, B. R., Jr., Beach, D., and Draetta, G. (1989). A 60-kDa cdc2-associated polypeptide complexes with the E1A proteins in adenovirus-infected cells. *Cell* **58,** 981–990.

Herskowitz, I. (1989). A regulatory hierarchy for cell specialization in yeast. *Nature (London)* **342,** 749–757.

Hu, Q., Bautista, C., Edwards, G., Defeo-Jones, D., Jones, R., and Harlow, E. (1991a). Antibodies specific for the human retinoblastoma protein identify a family of related polypeptides. Submitted for publication.

Hu, Q., Lees, J., Buchkovich, K., and Harlow, E. (1991b). The retinoblastoma protein associates with the human cdc2 kinase. Submitted for publication.

Huang, S., Lee, W.-H., and Lee, E. Y.-H. (1991). A cellular protein that competes with SV40 T antigen for binding to the retinoblastoma gene product. *Nature (London)* **350,** 160–162.

Kaelin, W. G., Pallas, D. C., DeCaprio, J. A., Kaye, F. J., and Livingston, D. M. (1991). Identification of cellular proteins that can interact specifically with the T/E1A-binding region of the retinoblastoma gene product. *Cell* **64,** 521–532.

Kinzler, K. W., Nilbert, M. C., Vogelstein, B., Bryan, T. M., Levy, D. B., Smith, K. J., Preisinger, A. C., Hamilton, S. R., Hedge, P., Markham, A., Carlson, M., Joslyn, G., Groden, J., White, R., Miki, Y., Miyoshi, Y., Nishisho, I., and Nakamura, Y. (1991). Identification of a gene located at chromosome 5q21 that is mutated in colorectal cancers. *Science* **251,** 1366–1370.

Lees, J., Buchkovich, K., Binns, G., Anderson, C., Marshak, D., and Harlow, E. (1991). The retinoblastoma protein is phosphorylated on multiple sites by human cdc2. Submitted for publication.

Ludlow, J. W., DeCaprio, J. A., Huang, C.-M., Lee, W.-H., Paucha, E., and Livingston, D. M. (1989). SV40 large T antigen binds preferentially to an underphosphorylated member of the retinoblastoma susceptibility gene product family. *Cell* **56,** 57–65.

Ludlow, J. W., Shon, J., Pipas, J. M., Livingston, D. M., and DeCaprio, J. A. (1990). The retinoblastoma susceptibility gene product undergoes cell cycle-dependent dephosphorylation and binding to and release from SV40 large T. *Cell* **60,** 387–396.

Marshall, C. J. (1991). Tumor suppressor genes. *Cell* **64,** 313–326.
Mihara, K., Cao, X.-R., Yen, A., Chandler, S., Driscoll, B., Murphree, A. L., T'Ang, A., and Fung, Y.-K. T. (1989). Cell cycle-dependent regulation of phosphorylation of the human retinoblastoma gene product. *Science* **246,** 1300–1303.
Rauscher, F., Morris, J., Tournay, D., Cook, D., and Curran, T. (1991). Binding of the Wilms' tumor locus zinc-finger protein to the EGR-1 consensus sequence. *Science* **250,** 1259–1262.
Roberts, A. B., and Sporn, M. B. (1990). *Handb. Exp. Pharmacol.* **95,** 419–472.
Rose, E. A., Glaser, T., Jones, C., Smith, C. L., Lewis, W. H., Call, K. M., Minden, M., Champagne, E., Bonetta, L., Yeger, H., and Housman, D. E. (1990). Complete physical map of the WAGR region of 11p13 localizes a candidate Wilms' tumor gene. *Cell* **60,** 495–508.
Wallace, M. R., Marchuk, D. A., Andersen, L. B., Letcher, R., Odeh, H. M., Saulino, A. M., and Fountain, J. W. (1990). Type 1 neurofibromatosis gene: Identification of a large transcript disrupted in three NF1 patients. *Science* **249,** 181–186.
Whyte, P., Buchkovich, J. J., Horowitz, J. M., Friend, S. H., Raybuck, M., Weinberg, R. A., and Harlow, E. (1988). Association between an oncogene and an antioncogene: The adenovirus E1A proteins bind to the retinoblastoma gene product. *Nature (London)* **334,** 124–129.
Xu, G., O'Connell, P., Viskochil, D., Cawthon, R., Robertson, M., Culver, M., Dunn, D., Stevens, J., Gesteland, R., White, R., and Weiss, R. (1990). The neurofibromatosis type 1 gene encodes a protein related to GAP. *Cell* **62,** 599–608.

8

Cellular Proteins That Can Interact Specifically with the Retinoblastoma Susceptibility Gene

WILLIAM G. KAELIN, JR.*, DAVID C. PALLAS*,
JAMES A. DeCAPRIO*, FREDERIC J. KAYE,†
AND DAVID M. LIVINGSTON*,

**The Dana-Farber Cancer Institute*
and Harvard Medical School
Boston, Massachusetts

†National Cancer Institute-Navy Medical Oncology Branch
and Uniformed Services, University of the Health Sciences
Bethesda, Maryland

I. Introduction

Inactivation of both copies of the retinoblastoma susceptibility gene (*RB-1*) has occurred in all sporadic and hereditary retinoblastomas examined to date. In addition, abnormalities involving the *RB-1* gene have been described in a variety of other human malignancies including small-cell lung carcinoma, osteosarcoma, soft-tissue sarcomas, breast carcinoma, bladder carcinoma, and prostate carcinoma (Bookstein *et al.*, 1990; Friend *et al.*, 1987; Harbour *et al.*, 1988; Horowitz *et al.*, 1990; Horowitz *et al.*, 1989; Lee *et al.*, 1988; Reissmann *et al.*, 1989; T'Ang *et al.*, 1988; Toguchida *et al.*, 1989; Varley *et al.*, 1989; Weichselbaum *et al.*, 1988; Yokota *et al.*, 1988). Consistent with the notion that *RB-1* serves as a tumor suppressor, Lee and co-workers have demonstrated that reintroduction of a wild-type *RB-1* gene into transformed cells that have lost the ability to express a functional *RB-1* gene product can lead to a decrease in cell growth rate and a diminished ability to form tumors in nude mice (Bookstein *et al.*, 1990; Huang *et al.*, 1988). *RB-1* encodes a 928-amino acid nuclear protein (RB), which is ubiquitously expressed among human tissues (Lee *et al.*, 1987a; Lee *et al.*, 1987b). How RB serves to regulate growth and prevent tumor formation remains uncertain. RB can bind to DNA-cellulose (Lee *et al.*, 1987b), but at present there are no data to suggest that RB can recognize a specific DNA sequence. Additional clues as to how RB might function have come from the study of DNA tumor viruses.

In 1987 Harlow and co-workers reported that adenovirus E1A was able to form a specific complex with RB (Whyte *et al.*, 1988). Subsequently it was demonstrated that SV40 large T antigen (T) (DeCaprio *et al.*, 1988) and the human papillomavirus E7 (Dyson *et al.*, 1989b) could also bind to RB. Although these viruses are not thought to be related to one another, each of these proteins contains a short, homologous, colinear sequence that, based on mutational analysis and peptide-competition studies, is thought to serve as the RB-binding motif (DeCaprio *et al.*, 1989; Kaelin *et al.*, 1990; Jones *et al.*, 1990). These sequences, typified by the region in E1A designated CR2, are also known to play a role in the ability of these viral proteins to transform cells (Green, 1989; Lillie *et al.*, 1987; Moran and Mathews, 1987). Furthermore, mutations in these sequences that abrogate RB binding lead to an inability to transform cells and vice versa (DeCaprio *et al.*, 1988; Green, 1989; Jones *et al.*, 1990; Moran, 1988; Phelps *et al.*, 1988; Whyte *et al.*, 1989). This has led to the hypothesis that at least part of the transforming function of these viral proteins is a product of their ability to interfere with one or more aspects of RB function.

RB exists in both un(der)phosphorylated (pRB) and phosphorylated (pRB^{phos}) forms. In the G_1 phase of the cell cycle, RB is present exclusively as pRB (DeCaprio *et al.*, 1989; Buchkovich *et al.*, 1989; Chen *et al.*, 1989; Mihara *et al.*, 1989; Ludlow *et al.*, 1990), whereas in S, G_2, and most of M, cells contain exclusively pRB^{phos} (DeCaprio *et al.*, 1989). Pulse-chase experiments demonstrate that newly synthesized pRB is phosphorylated at or near the G_1/S boundary and is dephosphorylated in M (Ludlow *et al.*, 1990). This suggests that RB function may be regulated during the cell cycle. Furthermore, T can bind only to un(der)phosphorylated RB (i.e., pRB) (Ludlow *et al.*, 1989). This suggests that pRB carries out those elements of RB growth-suppressor function(s) that are perturbed by T. Since RB is a growth-suppressor element, we have hypothesized that pRB contributes to an exit block at the G_1/S boundary. This block could, in theory, be alleviated by T binding or by the action of the cellular kinase(s) that normally phosphorylates pRB.

We, and others, have shown that a region in RB spanning residues 379–792 is sufficient for binding to E1A or T and must be relatively intact for binding to occur (Hu *et al.*, 1990; Huang *et al.*, 1990; Kaelin *et al.*, 1990). Furthermore, as an isolated polypeptide, this region of RB contains sufficient structural information to distinguish between wild-type T and the T mutant, K1, and can interact, stably and specifically, with a 14-residue peptide containing all of the pRB-binding domain of T (DeCaprio *et al.*, 1989; Kaelin *et al.*, 1990). The K1 protein is defective both in RB binding and in transformation, by virtue of a single amino acid substitution ($glu_{107} \rightarrow lys$) within the sequence represented by this peptide (Chen and Paucha, 1990; DeCaprio *et al.*, 1988; Kaelin *et al.*, 1990; Kalderon and Smith, 1984). That a relatively large portion of the RB portion should interact in a highly specific manner with a short, colinear sequence found in a diverse group of viral transforming proteins is reminiscent of a receptor–ligand type of interaction. Furthermore, this region of RB can be predicted to encode a leucine zipper (Bernards *et al.*, 1989; Hong *et al.*, 1989; McGee *et al.*, 1989), a structural motif that might participate in protein–protein interactions. Finally, the study of human tumors has, thus far, shown that all spontaneously occurring loss of function, RB mutations, that result in the synthesis of stable proteins, map to this region (see Fig. 1) (Bookstein *et al.*, 1990; Horowitz *et al.*, 1990; Horowitz *et al.*, 1989; Kaye *et al.*, 1990; Shew *et al.*, 1990a; Shew *et al.*, 1990b). This led us to hypothesize that RB function might be dependent on its ability to bind to a cellular protein (or proteins) bearing a sequence similar to that employed by E1A, T, and/or E7. Previous attempts to identify such a protein by coimmunoprecipitiation were, however, unsuccessful. We therefore devel-

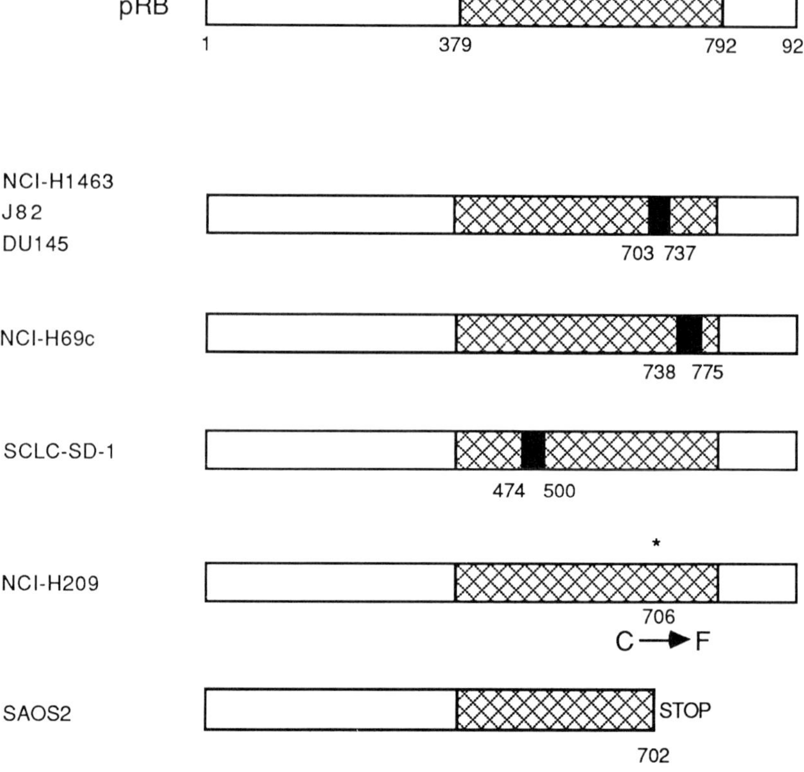

Fig. 1. Stable RB mutant proteins. Cell lines that express the various RB mutants are indicated on the left. See text for references. ■, In-frame deletion.

oped an RB-ligand binding assay that would circumvent many of the difficulties inherent in the use of coimmunoprecipitation, while enabling us to explore the significance of the above-mentioned genetic data. The question at hand was whether cells contain RB-binding proteins that can interact, specifically, with the 379–792 T/E1A/E7-binding domain of RB.

II. Results

The strategy used to identify RB-binding proteins is shown schematically in Fig. 2. Using the polymerase chain reaction (PCR) (Saiki *et al.*, 1988) and the prokaryotic expression vector pGEX-2T (Smith and Johnson, 1988), we generated a series of fusion proteins contain-

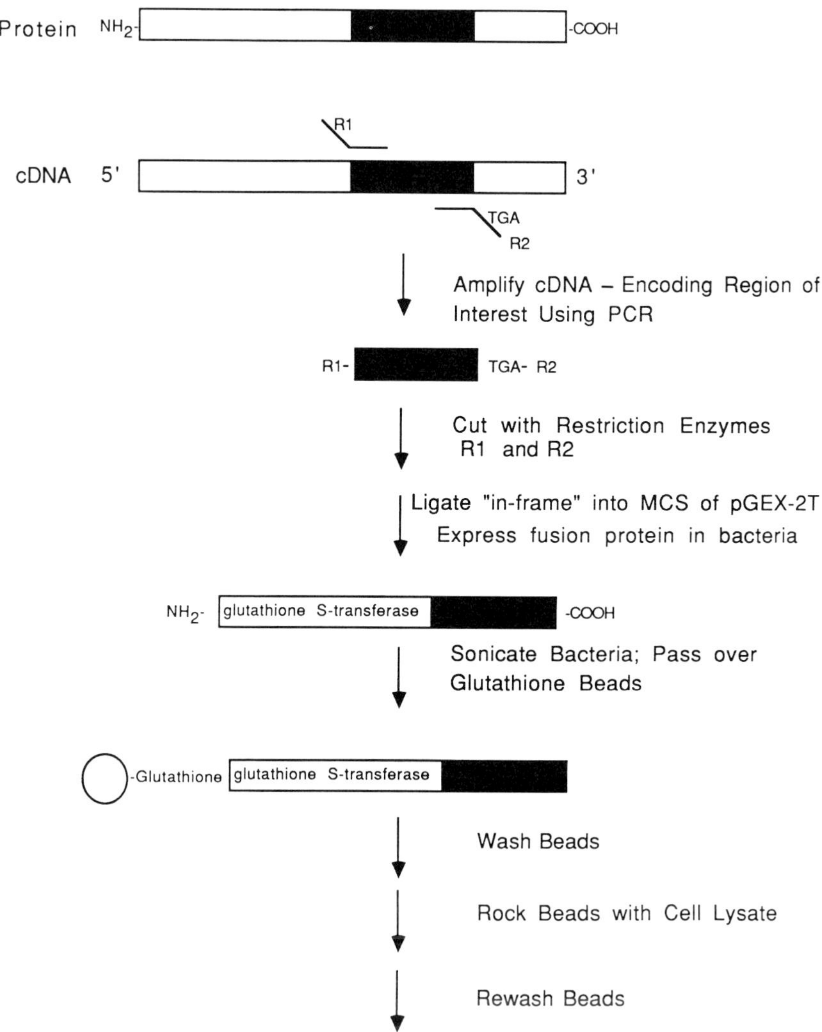

Fig. 2. Use of glutathione *S*-transferase fusion proteins to identify proteins capable of binding to a specific protein domain. R1 and R2 are restriction sites chosen to facilitate cloning into the multiple cloning site (MCS) of the prokaryotic expression vector pGEX-2T (Smith and Johnson, 1988).

ing an N-terminal glutathione *S*-transferase (GST) leader sequence and a C-terminal segment, which included either a mutant or intact version of the T/E1A-binding region of RB (see Fig. 3) (Kaelin *et al.*, 1991). Three of the fusion proteins [pGT-RB(379–928;dl Exon 21), pGT-RB(379–928;dl Exon 22), and pGT-RB(379–928;706 C $\rightarrow$ F)]

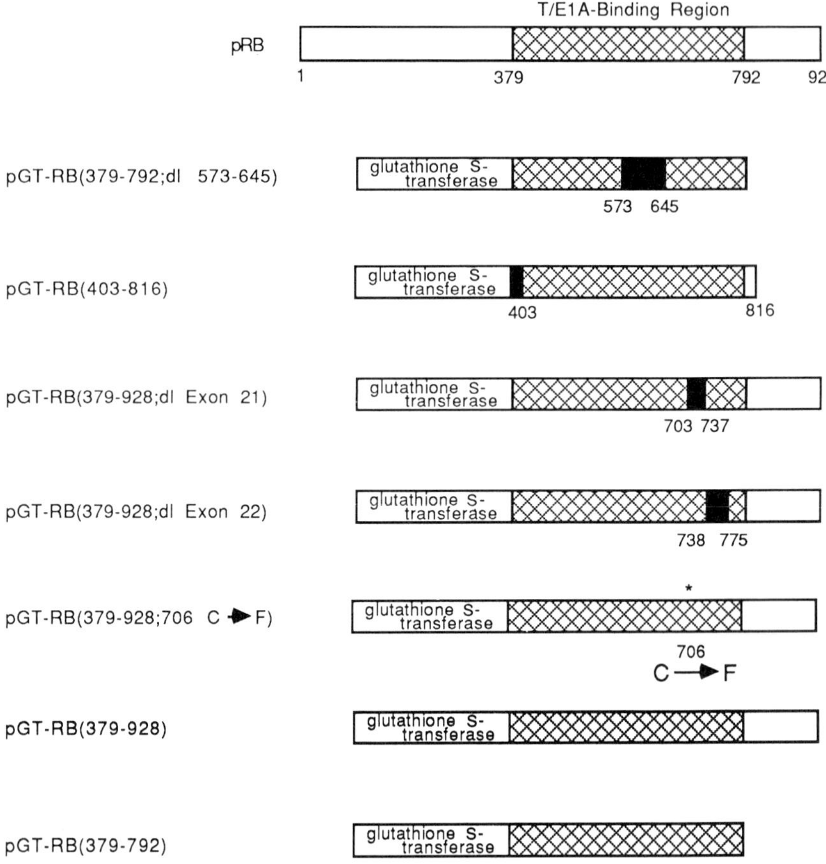

Fig. 3. Glutathione *S*-transferase/pRB fusion proteins. Reproduced from Kaelin *et al.* (1991) with permission of the publisher. ■, In-frame deletion.

contained mutations that correspond to naturally occuring RB mutations (compare with Fig. 1). Two of the fusion proteins contained intact replicas of the T/E1A-binding region, namely, pGT-RB(379–792) and pGT-RB(379–928).

Fusion proteins containing the GST leader sequence can be recovered from bacteria under nondenaturing conditions by sonication in the presence of a mild detergent, followed by equilibration with glutathione sepharose beads, to which the GST moiety binds specifically and noncovalently (Smith and Johnson, 1988). After the beads were washed, each fusion protein was bound in relatively pure form, as determined by Coomassie blue staining (Kaelin *et al.*, 1991). Aliquots of beads loaded with a given GST-RB fusion protein were then used as solid-phase affinity reagents with which to search for cell-encoded RB-binding proteins.

In pilot experiments, we demonstrated that the two fusion proteins that contained intact replicas of the T/E1A-binding region bound specifically to T or E1A, whereas the mutant derivatives were, as predicted, inactive (Kaelin *et al.*, 1991). None of the fusion proteins bound to K1T. Thus, the binding function of the T/E1A-binding region was not grossly altered by fusion to a foreign N-terminal sequence.

We next used this panel of GST-RB fusion proteins to search for cellular proteins capable of binding to RB in a manner similar to that employed by the abovementioned viral proteins. An ^{35}S-methionine-labeled lysate was prepared from exponentially growing WERI-RB27 retinoblastoma cells. The cell lysate was first precleared by serial incubation with glutathione sepharose loaded with GST alone. Aliquots of the cleared extract were then incubated with glutathione sepharose loaded with the various GST-RB fusion proteins, as described. After washing, bound proteins were eluted by boiling in a sodium dodecyl sulfate (SDS)-containing buffer, resolved by electrophoresis in a SDS-polyacrylamide gel, and visualized by fluorography. A family of approximately seven proteins (Fig. 4A and data not shown) were detected, which bound only to the two fusion proteins that contained intact replicas of the T/E1A-binding region (Kaelin *et al.*, 1991). To test further whether these proteins bound to RB in manner similar to that employed by T and E1A, we synthesized two 14-amino acid peptides. The T peptide, spanning T antigen residues 102–115, corresponded to the pRB-binding motif found in T, described earlier. The second peptide, designated K1, was identical to the T peptide, save for a glutamic acid to lysine substitution at residue 107. This latter peptide contains the mutation found in K1T, a protein that, as described, is defective in both transformation and in RB binding. The T peptide blocked the ability of the above-mentioned cellular proteins to interact with the two *wild-type* GST-RB fusion proteins in a concentration-dependent manner, whereas the K1 peptide had no discernable effect (Fig. 4B and data not shown) (Kaelin *et al.*, 1991). Purified T also competed with these cellular proteins for binding to the fusion proteins (Fig. 4B).

These observations were not restricted to the use of extracts prepared from WERI-RB27 cells. Similar results were obtained when

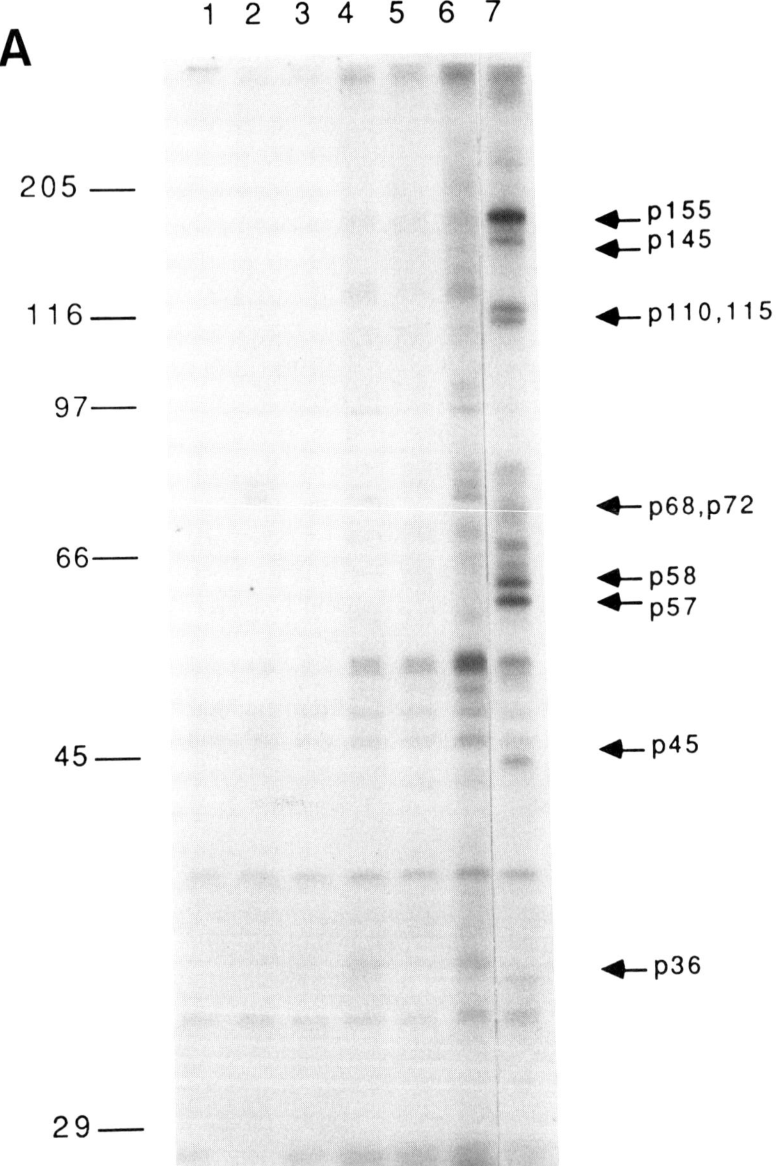

Fig. 4. Binding of cellular proteins to the pRB T/E1A-binding domain. (A) Aliquots of a metabolically labeled WERI-Rb27 cell lysate were incubated with glutathione sepharose (lane 1), or glutathione sepharose loaded with the pGEX-2T-encoded glutathione *S*-transferase leader sequence (lane 2); pGT-RB(379–792;dl 573-645) (lane 3); pGT-RB(403–816) (lane 4); pGT-RB(379–928;dl exon 21) (lane 5); pGT-RB(379–928;dl exon 22) (lane 6); or pGT-RB(379–

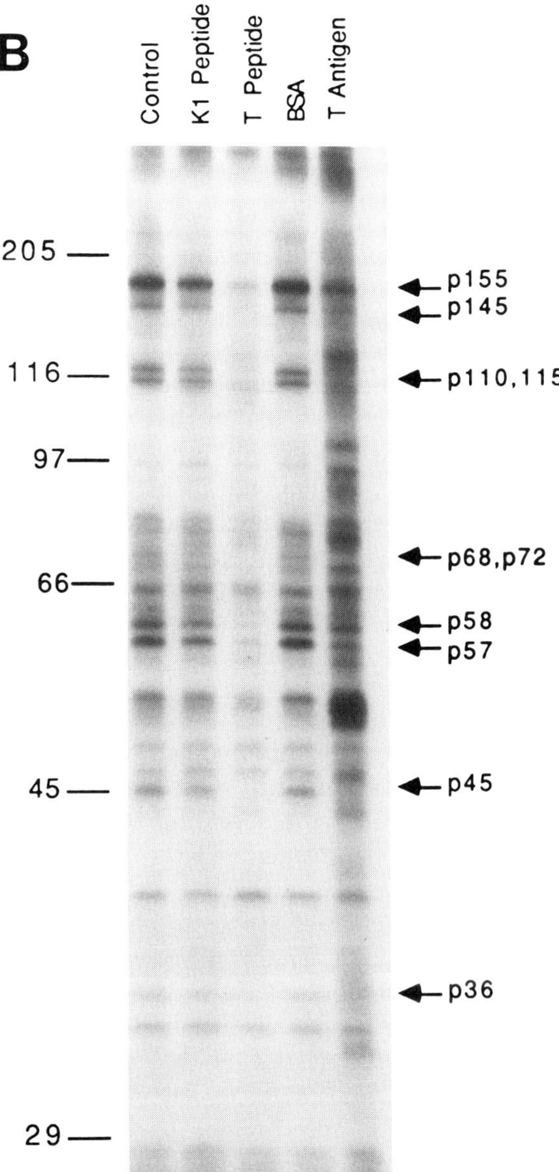

792) (lane 7). (B) Aliquots of precleared lysate were incubated with glutathione sepharose loaded with pGT-RB(379–792). pGT-RB(379–792) was blocked with 50 μg K1 peptide, 50 μg T peptide, 2 μg bovine serum albumin, or 2 μg purified T antigen before the addition of the cell lysate. Bound cellular proteins were resolved by electrophoresis and visualized by fluorography. Reproduced from Kaelin *et al.* (1991) with permission of the publisher.

extracts were prepared from the retinoblastoma cell lines, WERI-1 and RB 412, the bladder carcinoma line, J82, the prostate carcinoma line, DU145, the small-cell lung carcinoma line, NCI-H69c, and the osteosarcoma lines, SAOS2 and U2OS (Kaelin *et al.*, 1991). This latter cell line produces a functional RB-1 gene product (Lee *et al.*, 1987b); thus, synthesis of these candidate RB ligands is not peculiar to cells that have already mutated or lost both copies of *RB-1*.

Subcellular fractionation studies suggested that each of these candidate RB ligands was predominantly nuclear in location (Kaelin *et al.*, 1991). Cell-synchronization experiments demonstrated that the binding of one these proteins, p68-72, was enhanced when cell lysates from populations enriched in S-phase cells by hydroxyurea blockade were analyzed (Kaelin *et al.*, 1991). At the present time, we cannot determine whether this reflects an increase in the abundance of p68-72 during S phase, an increase in its affinity for RB during S phase, or both. Furthermore, we have not yet addressed the importance of RB phosphorylation on the binding of RB to any of the above-mentioned cellular proteins.

III. Discussion

Human cells contain a family of proteins that can bind, *in vitro*, to the T/E1A-binding region within RB. These proteins fail to bind RB targets bearing mutations corresponding to those found in spontaneously occurring, loss-of-function RB mutants. Furthermore, the binding of these proteins was abrogated or lost when reactions were carried out in the presence of synthetic peptides corresponding to sequences identified in E1A, T, and E7 as important for both transforming activity and RB binding. These data suggest that the binding of one or more of these proteins is essential for RB growth-suppression function(s). In the simplest of models, such a protein might, for example, help to provide a stimulus to cell growth when not bound to RB and lose that function once bound. Alternatively, one or more of these proteins might serve to regulate RB function in a positive fashion. Clearly multiple possibilities exist and, in the end, we must determine whether these proteins act *upstream* or *downstream* of RB in the maintenance of cell growth control.

The existence of candidate RB-binding proteins in nuclear extracts suggests that they might interact with RB *in vivo*. Experiments are in progress to test this hypothesis. Furthermore, the finding of enhanced binding during early S phase of p68-72 to RB is of potential interest, given the circumstantial evidence suggesting that RB contributes to a G_1 exit block.

RB is not the only host protein that forms a complex with T and E1A. In particular, two proteins, p300 and p107, both interact with these viral proteins in a manner similar to that employed by RB (DeCaprio *et al.,* 1989; Dyson *et al.,* 1989a; Ewen *et al.,* 1989; Whyte *et al.,* 1989; Morgan *et al.,* in preparation). In this regard, if we visualize the T/E1A-binding region within RB as a *pocket* that is recognized by sequences homologous to E1A CR2, then we can infer that p300 and p107 also contain such pockets. Therefore, the RB-binding proteins described here may be capable of interacting with one or both of these cellular proteins, as well. Conceivably, RB sequences outside the pocket region may determine whether a given RB-binding protein can in fact form a complex with each of these pocket proteins. Cloning of the genes for p300 and p107 should enable us to test these hypotheses.

We are currently performing experiments aimed at identifying the members of this new set of RB-binding proteins. We also wish to determine whether each of these proteins binds directly to RB or, alternatively, whether some bind indirectly, i.e., by "piggy-backing" to one, or perhaps a subset, of the RB-binding set. Ideally, understanding the identities and functions of these proteins will provide new insights into how RB regulates cell growth.

References

Bernards, R., Schackleford, G. M., Gerber, M. R., Horowitz, J. M., Friend, S. H., Schartl, M., Bogenmann, E., Rapaport, J. M., McGee, T., Dryja, T. P., and Weinberg, R. A. (1989). Structure and expression of the murine retinoblastoma gene and characterization of its encoded protein. *Proc. Natl. Acad. Sci. U.S.A.* **86,** 6474–6478.

Bookstein, R., Shew, J.-Y., Chen, P.-L., Scully, P., and Lee, W.-H. (1990). Suppression of tumorigenicity of human prostate carcinoma cells by replacing a mutated RB gene. *Science* **247,** 712–715.

Buchkovich, K., Duffy, L. A., and Harlow, E. (1989). The retinoblastoma protein is phosphorylated during specific phases of the cell cycle. *Cell* **58,** 1097–1105.

Chen, P., Scully, P.-L., Shew, J.-Y., Wang, J. Y. J., and Lee, W.-H. (1989). Phosphorylation of the retinoblastoma gene product is modulated during the cell cycle and cellular differentiation. *Cell* **58,** 1193–1198.

Chen, S., and Paucha, E. (1990). Identification of a region of simian virus 40 large T antigen required for cell transformation. *J. Virol.* **64,** 3350–3357.

DeCaprio, J. A., Ludlow, J. W., Figge, J., Shew, J.-Y., Huang, C.-M., Lee, W.-H., Marsilio, E., Paucha, E., and Livingston, D. M. (1988). SV40 large T antigen forms a specific complex with the product of the retinoblastoma susceptibility gene. *Cell* **54,** 275–283.

DeCaprio, J. A., Ludlow, J. W., Lynch, D., Furukawa, Y., Griffin, J., Piwnica-Worms, H., Huang, C.-M., and Livingston, D. M. (1989). The product of the retinoblastoma susceptibility gene has properties of a cell-cycle regulatory element. *Cell* **58,** 1085–1095.

Dyson, N., Buchkovich, K., Whyte, P., and Harlow, E. (1989a). The cellular 107K protein that binds to adenovirus E1A also associates with the large T antigens of SV40 and JC virus. *Cell* **58,** 249–255.

Dyson, N., Howley, P. M., Munger, K., and Harlow, E. (1989b). The human papilloma virus-16 E7 oncoprotein is able to bind to the retinoblastoma gene product. *Science* **243,** 934–937.

Ewen, M. E., Ludlow, J. W., Marsilio, E., Decaprio, J. A., Millikan, R. C., Cheng, S. H., Paucha, E., and Livingston, D. M. (1989). An N-terminal transformation-governing sequence of SV40 large T antigen contributes to the binding of both p110RB and a second cellular protein, p120. *Cell* **58,** 257–267.

Friend, S. H., Horowitz, J. M., Gerber, M. R., Wang, X., Bogenmann, E., Li, F. P., and Weinberg, R. A. (1987). Deletions of a DNA sequence in retinoblastomas and mesenchymal tumors: Organization of the sequence and its encoded protein. *Proc. Natl. Acad. Sci. U.S.A.* **84,** 9059–9063.

Green, M. R. (1989). When the products of oncogenes and antioncogenes meet. *Cell* **56,** 1–3.

Harbour, J. W., Lai, S., Whang-Peng, J., Gazdar, A. F., Minna, J. D., and Kaye, F. J. (1988). Abnormalities in structure and expression of the human retinoblastoma gene in SCLC. *Science* **241,** 353–356.

Hong, F. D., Huang, H.-S., To, H., Young, L.-S., Oro, A., Bookstein, R., Lee, E. Y.-H. P., and Lee, W.-H. (1989). Structure of the human retinoblastoma gene. *Proc. Natl. Acad. Sci. U.S.A.* **86,** 5502–5506.

Horowitz, J. M., Park, S.-H., Bogenmann, E., Cheng, J.-C., Yandell, D. W., Kaye, F. J., Minna, J. D., Dryja, T. P., and Weinberg, R. A. (1990). Frequent inactivation of the retinoblastoma antioncogene is restricted to a subset of human tumor cells. *Proc. Natl. Acad. Sci. U.S.A.* **87,** 2775–2779.

Horowitz, J. M., Yandell, D. W., Park, S.-H., Canning, S., Whyte, P., Buchkovich, K., Harlow, E., Weinberg, R. A., and Dryja, T. P. (1989). Point mutational inactivation of the retinoblastoma antioncogene. *Science* **243,** 937–940.

Hu, Q., Dyson, N., and Harlow, E. (1990). The regions of the retinoblastoma protein needed for binding to adenovirus E1A or SV40 large T antigen are common sites for mutations. *EMBO J.* **9,** 1147–1155.

Huang, H.-J. S., Yee, J.-K., Shew, J.-Y., Chen, P.-L., Bookstein, R., Friedmann, T., Lee, E. Y.-H. P., and Lee, W.-H. (1988). Suppression of the neoplastic phenotype by replacement of the RB gene in human cancer cells. *Science* **242,** 1563–1566.

Huang, H.-J. S., Wang, N.-P., Tseng, B. Y., Lee, W. -H., and Lee, E. Y.-H. P. (1990). Two distinct and frequently mutated regions of retinoblastoma protein are required for binding to SV40 T antigen. *EMBO J.* **9,** 1815–1822.

Jones, R. E., Wegrzyn, R. J., Patrick, D. R., Balishin, N. L., Vuocolo, G. A., Riemen, M. W., Defeo-Jones, D., Garsky, V. M., Heimbrook, D. C., and Oliff, A. (1990). Identification of HPV-16 E7 peptides that are potent antagonists of E7 binding to the retinoblastoma suppressor protein. *J. Biol. Chem.* **265,** 12782–12785.

Kaelin, W. G., Ewen, M. E., and Livingston, D. M. (1990). Definition of the minimal simian virus 40 large T antigen- and adenovirus E1A-binding domain in the retinoblastoma gene product. *M.C.B.* **10,** 3761–3769.

Kaelin, W. G., Pallas, D. C., DeCaprio, J. A., Kaye, F. J., and Livingston, D. M. (1991). Identification of cellular proteins which can interact specifically with the T/E1A-binding region of the retinoblastoma susceptibility gene product. *Cell* **64,** 521–532.

Kalderon, D., and Smith, A. E. (1984). *In vitro* mutagenesis of a putative DNA-binding domain of SV40 large-T. *Virology* **139,** 109–137.

Kaye, F. J., Kratzke, R. A., Gerster, J. L., and Horowitz, J. M. (1990). A single amino acid substitution results in a retinoblastoma protein defective in phosphorylation and oncoprotein binding. *Proc. Natl. Acad. Sci. U.S.A.* **87,** 6922–6926.

Lee, E. Y.-H. P., To, H., Dhew, J.-Y., Bookstein, R., Scully, P., and Lee, W.-H. (1988). Inactivation of the retinoblastoma susceptibility gene in human breast cancers. *Science* **241,** 218–221.

Lee, W.-H., Bookstein, R., Hong, F., Young, L.-J., Shew, J.-Y., and Lee, E. Y.-H. P. (1987a). Human retinoblastoma susceptibility gene: Cloning, identification, and sequence. *Science* **235,** 1394–1399.

Lee, W.-H., Shew, J.-Y., Hong, F. D. Sery, T. W., Donoso, L. A., Young, L.-J., Bookstein, R., and Lee, E. Y.-H. P. (1987b). The retinoblastoma susceptibility gene encodes a nuclear phosphoprotein associated with DNA binding activity. *Nature (London)* **329,** 642–645.

Lillie, J. W., Loewenstein, P. M., Green, M. R., and Green, M. (1987). Functional domains of adenovirus type 5 E1a proteins. *Cell* **50,** 1091–1100.

Ludlow, J. W., DeCaprio, J. A., Huang, C.-M., Lee, W.-H., Paucha, E., and Livingston, D. M. (1989). SV40 Large T antigen binds preferentially to an underphosphorylated member of the retinoblastoma susceptibility gene product family. *Cell* **56,** 57–65.

Ludlow, J. W., Shon, J., Pipas, J. M., Livingston, D. M., and Decaprio, J. A. (1990). The retinoblastoma susceptibility gene product undergoes cell cycle-dependent dephosphorylation and binding to and release from SV40 large T. *Cell* **60,** 387–396.

McGee, T. L., Yandell, D. W., and Dryja, T. P. (1989). Structure and partial genomic sequence of the human retinoblastoma susceptibility gene. *Gene* **80,** 119–128.

Mihara, K., Cao, X.-R., Yen, A., Chandler, S., Driscoll, B., Murphree, A. L., T'Ang, A., and Fung, Y.-K. T. (1989). Cell cycle-dependent regulation of phosphorylation of the human retinoblastoma gene product. *Science* **246,** 1300–1303.

Moran, E. (1988). A region of SV40 large T antigen can substitute for a transforming domain of the adenovirus E1A products. *Nature (London)* **334,** 168–170.

Moran, E., and Mathews, M. B. (1987). Multiple functional domains in the adenovirus E1A gene. *Cell* **48,** 177–178.

Phelps, W. C., Yee, C. L., Munger, K., and Howley, P. M. (1988). The human papillomavirus type 16 E7 gene encodes transactivation and transformation functions similar to those of adenovirus E1A. *Cell* **53,** 539–547.

Reissmann, P. T., Simon, M. A., Lee, W.-H., and Slamon, D. J. (1989). Studies of the retinoblastoma gene in human sarcomas. *Oncogene* **4**, 839–843.

Saiki, R. K., Gelfand, D. H., Stoffel, S., Scharf, S. J., Higuchi, R., Horn, G. T., Mullis, K. B., and Erlich, H. A. (1988). Primer-directed enzymatic amplification of DNA with a thermostable DNA polymerase. *Science* **239**, 487–491.

Shew, J.-Y., Chen, P.-L., Bookstein, R., Lee, E. Y.-H. P., and Lee, W.-H. (1990a). Deletion of a splice donor site ablates expression of the following exon and produces an unphosphorylated RB protein unable to bind SV40 T antigen. *Cell Growth and Differentiation* **1**, 17–25.

Shew, J.-Y., Lin, B. T.-Y., Chen, P.-L., Tseng, B. Y., Yang-Feng, T. L., and Lee, W.-H. (1990b). C-terminal truncation of the retinoblastoma gene product leads to functional inactivation. *Proc. Natl. Acad. Sci. U.S.A.* **87**, 6–10.

Smith, D. B., and Johnson, K. S. (1988). Single-step purification of polypeptides expressed in *Escherichia coli* as fusions with glutathione S-transferase. *Gene* **67**, 31–40.

T'Ang, A., Varley, J. M., Chakraborty, S., Murphree, A. L., and Fung, Y.-K. T. (1988). Structural rearrangement of the retinoblastoma gene in human breast cancer. *Science* **242**, 263–266.

Toguchida, J., Ishizaki, K., Sasaki, M. S., Nakamura, Y., Ikenaga, M., Kato, M., Sugimot, M., Kotoura, Y., and Yamamuro, T. (1989). Preferential mutation of paternally derived RB gene as the initial event in sporadic osteosarcoma. *Nature (London)* **338**, 156–158.

Varley, J. M., Armour, J., Swallow, J. E., Jeffreys, A. J., Ponder, B. A. J., T'Ang, A., Fung, Y.-K. T., Brammar, W. J., and Walker, R. A. (1989). The retinoblastoma gene is frequently altered leading to loss of expression in primary breast tumours. *Oncogene* **4**, 725–729.

Weichselbaum, R. R., Beckett, M., and Diamond, A. (1988). Some retinoblastomas, osteosarcomas, and soft-tissue sarcomas may share a common etiology. *Proc. Natl. Acad. Sci. U.S.A.* **85**, 2106–2109.

Whyte, P., Buchkovich, K. J., Horowitz, J. M., Friend, S. H., Raybuck, M., Weinberg, R. A., and Harlow, E. (1988). Association between an oncogene and an antioncogene: The adenovirus E1A proteins bind to the retinoblastoma gene product. *Nature (London)* **334**, 124–129.

Whyte, P., Williamson, N. M., and Harlow, E. (1989). Cellular targets for transformation by the adenovirus E1A proteins. *Cell* **56**, 67–75.

Yokota, J., Akiyama, T., Fung, Y.-K. T., Benedict, W. F., Namba, Y., Hanaoka, M., Wada, M., Terasaki, T., Shimosato, Y., Sugimura, T., and Terada, M. (1988). Altered expression of the retinoblastoma (RB) gene in small-cell lung carcinoma of the lung. *Oncogene* **3**, 471–475.

9

Role of the Wilms' Tumor 1 Tumor-Suppressor Gene in the Etiology of Wilms' Tumor

DAVID E. HOUSMAN

Center for Cancer Research
Massachusetts Institute of Technology
Cambridge, Massachusetts

I. Introduction

The role that tumor-suppressor genes play in the development of human cancers is clearly a significant but as yet largely uncharted area of cancer research. This chapter will focus on Wilms' tumor (WT), a childhood malignancy derived from embryonal kidney cells. I hope, however, to place recent progress in the understanding of WT into the broader framework of understanding the significance of tumor-suppressor genes in the etiology of human cancer.

A. What Are Tumor-Suppressor Genes?

Tumor-suppressor genes may be defined in the broadest sense as the group of genes for which gene inactivation contributes to the unregulated proliferation of the cells. Two basic lines of evidence led to this concept. First, somatic cell hybridization experiments demonstrated that fusion between tumor cells and normal cells led to hybrids that had a phenotype more closely like the normal cell parent than the tumor cell parent (Harris *et al.*, 1969). As chromosome segregation proceeded in such hybrids, the reemergence of the transformed phenotype could often be observed (Sager, 1985). In a number of specific instances, loss of growth control could be correlated with the absence of a specific chromosome derived from the normal parental cell (Sager, 1985). These results led to the inference that the normal cell contributed an active copy of a gene (the tumor-suppressor gene), which regulated the growth of the hybrid cell and hence suppressed its potential tumorigenicity (Harris *et al.*, 1969). The second line of evidence supporting the existence of tumor-suppressor genes came from analysis of specific childhood cancers, with particular attention to the age of onset and the number of tumors per individual. In an analysis of retinoblastoma, Knudson was able to demonstrate that children with a hereditary predisposition to this eye tumor showed an early age of onset and a distribution in the number of tumors per individual that was mathematically most compatible with a single rate-limiting hit (Knudson, 1971). Children with sporadic retinoblastoma on the other hand, showed a later and only a single tumor per individual, at age of onset, consistent with two rate-limiting hits. A parallel analysis with similar conclusions was carried out by Knudson and Strong for Wilms' tumor (1972). These analyses were subsequently interpreted to indicate that the rate-limiting events in the formation of a retinoblastoma or a Wilms' tumor are the loss of function of both copies of a key tumor-suppressor gene. In hereditary cases, one copy of the tumor-suppressor gene was presumably inactivated by a germline mutation. The loss of the second copy by a somatic event (mutation, nondisjunction or mitotic crossing over) would be the single rate-limiting event in hereditary tumors. Sporadic tumors would, according to this analysis, result from the occurrence of a somatic event (point mutation or deletion) inactivating one of the two homologs of a tumor-suppressor gene, followed by a second somatic event inactivating the second copy of the gene, thus giving rise to a cell in which the tumor-suppressor gene was functionally inactive. It is important to note that the Knudson hit-kinetics analysis applied primarily to childhood cancers, while the somatic cell genetic technique provided support for the relevance of tumor-suppressor genes in adult cancers as well. While both lines of evidence provided direct support for the existence of tumor-suppressor genes, precise identification of the relevant genes has involved a series of complementary experimental strategies.

B. Locating and Isolating Tumor-Suppressor Genes

The identification of tumor-suppressor genes has been a formidable task. The isolation and characterization of positive oncogenes, a class of genes that play an important role in regulating cell proliferation, proceeded by a direct route. Because oncogenes act by providing cells with the ability to circumvent normal growth regulation by the introduction of a new function into the cell, they can be assayed directly, via DNA or viral transformation. In contrast, the genetic strategies that have led to the isolation of tumor-suppressor genes have, (with one exception, p53), taken a less direct strategy, utilizing gene-mapping techniques. Several genetic strategies have contributed to the isolation of tumor-suppressor genes. First, as noted above, the inactivation of a tumor-suppressor gene may involve loss of the normal copy of the gene via a chromosomal event, nondisjunction, or mitotic crossing over. The occurrence of such events can be assayed by the loss of heterozygosity of polymorphic DNA markers on the chromosome carrying the tumor-suppressor gene. In each case in which inactivation of a tumor-suppressor gene has been associated with a specific tumor type, an increased frequency of loss of heterozygosity has been observed for the chromosome carrying the tumor-suppressor gene compared to other chromosomes in the tumor. Loss of heterozygosity is therefore considered to be a significant clue in the search for a tumor-suppressor gene. However, loss-of-heterozygosity studies do have limitations and pitfalls. Whereas in most childhood cancers, the karyotype may remain near normal, in adult cancers karyotypic instability in the tumor cells can be extreme. In one study of metastatic melanomas, as many as 25% of the DNA markers assayed had lost heterozygosity (Dracopoli *et al.*, 1987). While it is possible that all of the karyotypic changes that occur in these tumors relate directly to meaningful losses in gene function in the tumor cells, this is by no means certain. The significance of loss of heterozygosity in the context of such extreme karyotypic instability must thus be considered carefully. A further limitation of loss of heterozygosity studies is the likelihood that they can give at best only an approximation of the position of the relevant tumor-suppressor gene. Loss of heterozygosity due to chromosomal nondisjunction can provide support for the localization of a tumor-suppressor gene to a specific chromosome, but provides no information as to where on that chromosome the tumor-suppressor gene may lie. Mitotic recombination, or other mechanisms involving partial chromosome loss, can be more informative. The location of the chromosome segment that most frequently demonstrates loss of heterozygosity can thus be a clue to the location of the tumor-suppressor gene; however, such data do not necessarily provide a precise localization of the gene involved. Another approach that can potentially give information on the position of a tumor-suppressor gene is the analysis of families that show inherited predisposition for a given cancer or set of cancers using genetic-linkage techniques. While this approach has been particularly valuable in relating the contribution of genes isolated by other techniques to familial cancer, the precision of linkage analysis is also not high in locating specific genes unless very large numbers of genetically homogeneous families are available. To date, the most powerful discriminator of the position of a tumor-suppressor gene has been the identification and analysis of internal chromosome deletions. Chromosomal deletions that have contributed to the identification of tumor-suppressor genes occur in two contexts. Deletions of a chromosome segment that includes a tumor-suppressor gene can and do occur during gametogenesis. A sperm or egg carrying such a deletion can thus contribute an incomplete set of genetic instructions to the embryo, resulting in hemizygosity for all the genes within the deleted chromosomal segment, including the tumor-suppressor gene. A child carrying such a deletion falls into the *one-hit* category of Knudson, and is thus likely to have multiple tumors of independent origin. Children with multiple Wilms' tumors or multiple retinoblastoma tumors associated with hemizygosity of specific chromosomal segments in all tissues have been identified in the clinical literature for more than a decade (Yunis and Ramsey, 1978; Riccardi *et al.*, 1978). In addition to the development of tumors, these children often exhibit multiple congenital malformations leading to ready recognition in the clinic. The germline karyotypic abnormalities in these children are quite specific, in contrast to the more disorderly karyotypic picture observed even in the tumors themselves. Analysis of the deletions from a series of such children has helped to define the location of genes for both retinoblastoma and Wilms' tumor. However, while this approach for localization of tumor-suppressor genes provides higher definition than methods discussed previously, the deletions observed are quite large and can usually be measured in megabases. To further localize a tumor-suppressor gene, much smaller deletions are required. Such deletions can and do occur in sporadic tumors at a measurable frequency for both retinoblastoma and Wilms' tumor. Of particular value are tumors in which both copies of the tumor-suppressor gene have been lost by deletion, a situation referred to as homozygous deletion. For both retinoblastoma and Wilms' tumor, the frequency of tumors carrying homozygous deletion appears to be between 1 in 50 and 1 in 100. Tumors of this type are particularly valuable in pinpointing the location of the retinoblastoma (Dryja *et al.*, 1986) and Wilms' tumor (Lewis *et al.*, 1988) genes to within a few hundred kb, as well as identifying the location of the deleted in colon carcinoma (DCC) tumor-suppressor gene, which contributes to the etiology of adult colon cancer (Fearon *et al.*, 1990).

Once a candidate transcription unit has been identified within the region of homozygous deletion, the definitive identification of the tumor-suppressor gene can be still be a challenging task. Two strategies have been taken to date: First, analysis of a series of tumors that have undergone homozygous deletion can limit the smallest region of overlap to the candidate transcription unit. Second, inactivating point mutations, small deletions, or rearrangements can be demonstrated within the coding region of the gene itself for both sporadic tumors and germline mutations in hereditary cases.

II. The Genetics of Wilms' Tumor

A. Identification of the WT1 Gene

The experimental route that has led to the isolation of a tumor-suppressor gene for Wilms' tumor followed the pathway has been outlined. The first evidence that Wilms' tumor can be associated with a specific set of congenital abnormalities was a 1964 study by Miller, Fraumeni, and Manning (Miller *et al.*, 1964), which demonstrated that Wilms' tumor can be found in association with a characteristic constellation of symptoms that came to be termed the WAGR syndrome. This symptom group includes Wilms' tumor, often in a bilateral form, aniridia (absence or malformation of the iris), genitourinary malformations, and mental retardation. Subsequent karyotypic analysis led to the identification of constitutional deletions of the short arm of chromosome 11, which (although of varying sizes) invariably included deletion of at least a portion of band 11p13. These studies led to the inference that a tumor-suppressor gene for Wilms' tumor was located in this chromosome band in the immediate proximity of genes responsible for the other phenotypes of the WAGR syndrome. Isolation and characterization of large numbers of anonymous DNA sequences from the short arm of chromosome 11 led to the eventual isolation of a number of clones, which not only were hemizygously deleted in the germline of all WAGR patients examined, but also identified a segment of homozygous deletion in a number of sporadic Wilms' tumors (Call *et al.*, 1990; Gessler *et al.*, 1990; Lewis *et al.*, 1988; Rose *et al.*, 1990). These cloned DNA sequences in turn led to the definition of the transcription unit encoding the WT1 tumor-suppressor gene (Call *et al.*, 1990). This transcription unit encodes a zinc-finger polypeptide of approximately 50 kDa. The structural characteristics of the predicted polypeptide suggest that it is a sequence-specific DNA-binding protein that regulates transcription (Call *et al.*, 1990; Rausher *et al.*, 1990). In contrast to the ubiquitously expressed RB1 gene, the WT1 gene is expressed in a highly tissue-specific manner (Buckler *et al.*, 1991; Call *et al.*, 1990; Pritchard-Jones *et al.*, 1990). The embryonic kidneys and the urogenital system are the tissues that show highest expression levels of the WT1 gene (Buckler *et al.*, 1991; Call *et al.*, 1990; Pritchard-Jones *et al.*, 1990).

B. Evidence That the WT1 Gene Is the 11p13 Tumor-Suppressor Gene

A number of lines of evidence support the identification of WT1 as the 11p13 tumor-suppressor gene. The WT1 mRNA is encoded by a transcription unit that encompasses approximately 50 kbp (Call *et al.*, 1990). Some Wilms' tumors contain deletions that include this 50-kbp transcription unit along with adjacent genomic DNA sequences (Call *et al.*, 1990; Gessler *et al.*, 1990). However, tumors have been identified in which the region of homozygous deletion includes only a portion of the WT transcription unit. Tumors that show homozygous deletion extending into the upstream exons (Ton *et al.*, in press) or into the downstream exons of the WT transcription unit (Cowell *et al.*, submitted) have now been described. These results taken together define the smallest region of overlap of homozygous 11p13 deletions in Wilms' tumor to be within the genomic DNA segment that encodes the WT1 gene. Small internal deletions that directly alter mRNA structure have also been identified within the WT1 transcription unit in Wilms' tumors (Haber *et al.*, 1990; Huff *et al.*, 1991; Pelletier *et al.*, submitted). In at least two instances, the internal deletion leads to premature chain termination of the WT1 polypeptide. In most of these cases, chromosome 11 has undergone either non-disjunction or mitotic recombination during tumorigenesis so that only the mutant copy of the WT1 gene is present in the tumor. The findings in these Wilms' tumors thus indicate that complete loss of function of the WT1 gene is consistent with Wilms' tumorigenesis and support the identification of this transcription unit and its gene product as the 11p13 Wilms' tumor gene.

C. Complete Loss of Function of the WT1 Gene May Not Be Required for Wilms' Tumorigenesis

Complete loss of function of the WT1 gene may not be the only route to Wilms' tumor. At least one mutation in a Wilms' tumor has the characteristics of a so-called dominant negative mutation. A 25-bp deletion at the 3′ splice junction of exon 9 causes the removal of the nucleotide sequences encoding exon 9 from the WT1 mRNA to yield an in-frame deletion (Haber *et al.*, 1990). The polypeptide encoded by this mRNA is predicted to be lacking zinc-finger 3. This polypeptide fails to bind DNA within sequence specificity (Rausher *et al.*, 1990) but may still interact competitively with protein targets of the WT1 polypeptide, allowing the mutated gene product to competitively inhibit function of the wild-type WT1 product. Another possibility that should be considered for WT1 is that a threshold effect may govern the effectiveness of the WT1 gene product in carrying out its normal functions. A significant reduction in the level of an otherwise normal WT1 gene product could thus be a decisive event in the formation of some Wilms' tumors.

D. WT Genes at Other Genetic Locations

As discussed, the relationship between the WT1 gene and the etiology of at least a proportion of Wilms' tumors is clear. However, there is evidence that genes located at two other chromosomal sites can play an important role in the etiology of Wilms' tumor. Wilms' tumor is found in association with a second rare clinical condition, Beckwith-Wiedemann syndrome (BWS), whose clinical features are quite distinct from those of the WAGR syndrome (Sotelo-Avila *et al.*, 1980). A fraction of BWS cases show rearrangement (generally duplication) of band p15 of chromosome 11 (Waziri *et al.*, 1983). On the other hand, band p13 is found to be intact in these patients (Glaser *et al.*, 1990). These results suggest that a locus in band p15 is involved in the etiology of Wilms' tumor, at least in some cases. The existence of this second locus is also supported by loss-of-heterozygosity (LOH) studies, which demonstrate allelic losses for markers restricted to 11p15 in about 15% of Wilms' tumor cases (Koufos *et al.*, 1989; Reeve *et al.*, 1989). Mutations of loci in band 11p15 and 11p13 (WT1) may represent alternative pathways in Wilms' tumorigenesis. Alternatively, in some Wilms' tumors, inactivation of both loci may be required, as suggested by some patients with WAGR syndrome whose tumors show LOH restricted to 11p15. The assessment of the number of genes that may contribute to Wilms' tumorigenesis is further complicated by studies of rare families that show hereditary transmission of predisposition to Wilms' tumor. Linkage to markers in both 11p13 and 11p15 to predisposition to Wilms' tumor has been excluded in these studies, suggesting the existence of a third WT locus (Grundy *et al.*, 1988; Huff *et al.*, 1988; Schwartz *et al.*, submitted).

E. Characteristics of the WT1 Gene

Analysis of the expression pattern and deduced amino acid sequence of the WT1 gene suggests that the WT1 gene product is a transcription factor that regulates the program of differentiation of nephroblasts of the developing kidney. Two alternative splice choices occur in the synthesis of WT1 mRNA, leading to the production of four mRNAs and four corresponding polypeptides (Haber *et al.*, submitted). Within the amino terminal segment of each of the predicted polypeptides is an extremely proline-rich segment (11 of 12 amino acids in one segment are prolines in the human WT1 gene). This corresponds to a similar segment in exon 1 of the RB1 gene (Friend *et al.*, 1987; Lee *et al.*, 1987). The precise functional significance of the proline-rich domains is not yet established for either polypeptide. Proline-rich regions have been described for a number of transcription factors (see Mitchell and Tjian, 1989). The cellular targets of the non-zinc-finger portion of the WT polypeptide remain an area of intense interest. It seems reasonable to presume that the WT1 gene product interacts with other cellular factors that control transcription.

F. What Are the Normal Functions of the WT1 Gene?

WT1 has a limited pattern of tissue-specific expression. During mouse kidney development, WT1 expression peaks between days 17 *postcoitum* and days 3 *postpartum* (Buckler *et al.*, 1991). The highest expression levels for the WT1 gene are found during embryonic development and early neonatal life in the cells of the metanephric blastema. Within the developing kidney, *in situ* hybridization studies have shown WT1 expression to be highest in the cells destined to become glomeruli, the so-called S-shaped bodies (Pritchard-Jones, *et al.*, 1990; Zabel *et al.*, submitted). These observations suggest that the WT1 gene products play an important role in regulating both the proliferation and differentiation of these progenitor cells.

The WT1 gene is also expressed at high levels in the differentiating testes and ovaries (Pelletier *et al.*, submitted). In contrast to the kidney, expression in these organs continues at high levels throughout adult life. WT1 expression is observed at lower levels in a number of other adult organs, including spleen, heart, and lung (Call *et al.*, 1990; Buckler *et al.*, 1991). It seems reasonable to propose that in the developing nephroblast, the WT1 gene products play a central role in limiting the proliferation of cells that make up the differentiating glomerulus. The WT1 gene product may also regulate transcription to contribute to the initiation of the terminal stages of the differentiation program. Identification of genes for which transcription is directly controlled by WT1 would clearly be of great interest. What is the role of WT1 in the tissues of the genital system? The occurrence of developmental abnormalities of the urogenital system in the WAGR syndrome can be directly attributed to the effect of half-dosage of the WT1 gene products (Pelletier *et al.*, submitted). As in the kidney, WT1 is expressed in very specific cell types in the genital system and particularly in the female, at very discrete stages in the differentiation program. It is not unreasonable to presume that the transcriptional regulation of WT1 in the genital system also relates to controlling the balance between proliferation and differentiation. The physiological role of WT1 in spleen, heart, and lung remains an intriguing question at present. Unlike in the kidney and spleen, there are no clear-cut developmental abnormalities in these organs in WAGR patients or in patients with germline mutations in the WT1 gene. The role of the WT1 gene in the control of cellular phenotypes in these organs awaits additional observations and experimentation.

G. An Analog in the Mouse to Human WAGR Deletions

The development of mouse strains in which the WT1 gene is inactivated or overexpressed may give insight into the role of WT1 in tumorigenesis and development. Recently, we have described a deletion in the mouse that is genetically analogous to WAGR deletions in man (Glaser *et al.*, 1990). The Sey^{Dey} deletion mutation in the mouse encompasses the mouse homologs of the human chromosome 11p13 Wilms' tumor (WT1) (Buckler *et al.*, 1991) and aniridia (AN2) loci. Mice carrying the deletion, however, do not exhibit an increased frequency of nephroblastoma. This difference in phenotype between regions of synteny rendered hemizygous in mouse and man may result from a number of causes. The number of cells involved in the formation of the mouse kidney is much smaller than the corresponding cell number in man. If the frequency of events leading to tumor formation is the same in both species, then failure to detect tumors in the mouse might reflect the difference in the number of target cells. Alternatively, the difference between the two species may reflect a difference in the status of other genes required for malignant transformation of nephroblasts.

III. Comparison of Wilms' Tumor 1 to Other Tumor-Suppressor Genes

The WT1 gene is one of a small number of tumor-suppressor genes that have been definitively identified to date. These include RB1, p53, DCC, and NF1. One of the striking aspects of this list is that members of the group have diverse functional characteristics. RB1 and p53 appear to be nuclear factors that control transcription. Unlike WT1, neither RB1 nor p53 appears to have an obvious sequence-specific DNA-binding domain. DCC shows striking homology to the N-CAM and other genes involved in cell adhesion. NF1 has been shown to have homology to GAP proteins, indicating that it is likely to exert its effects on cellular proliferation through the RAS signal-transduction pathway. The diversity of modes of action of the known tumor-suppressor genes is complemented by the differences among the specificity of expression. RB1 and p53 are expressed in essentially all tissues examined, while WT1, NF1, and DCC show very clear differences in expression levels among different tissues and cell types. Given the diversity of functional characteristics and expression patterns, what common functional feature relates the tumor-suppressor genes?

One view of the problem is that any gene involved in the process of controlling the decisions of cells to divide or differentiate has the potential to be a tumor-suppressor gene. However, the number of such genes must be quite large. Can every gene that plays a role in regulating such decisions be a tumor-suppressor gene? There is a good reason to believe that this may not be the case. If the frequency of inactivation of a gene during the lifetime of an organism approaches the number of cells present in the body that will give rise to a tumor if that gene is inactivated, then the occurrence of a potentially life-threatening tumor is close to a certainty. This is precisely the situation that occurs when there has been a germline mutation in the RB1 gene. The reproductive fitness of an organism carrying such an inactivating mutation is extremely low, if the cancer occurs before or during the reproductively active portion of the life cycle. For this reason, it is unlikely that there are a large number of situations analogous to retinoblastoma, Wilms' tumor, and Li-Fraumeni syndrome (germline inactivation of the p53 gene) in which a single gene inactivation is rate limiting to the occurrence of the tumor. It seems more likely that pathways to tumorigenesis involving multiple rate-limiting gene inactivations of about equal probability will be the rule rather than the exception. Indeed, somatic inactivation of the RB1 and p53 genes are likely to be important in a number of tumor types (small-cell lung cancer, breast, bladder, sarcoma) in which the inactivation of one of these genes alone is not sufficient to cause tumorigeneis.

IV. Implications in the Search for Tumor-Suppressor Genes for Adult Cancers

The search for tumor-suppressor genes is an essential component to understanding the pathways involved in tumorigenesis. The lessons learned in the searches that have been successful thus far should be considered in the design of searches for new tumor-suppressor genes. The strategy utilized to isolate the RB1 and WT1 genes is particularly well suited to the childhood cancers, in which large constitutional deletions pinpoint the chromosomal region within which the search for homozygous deletions is likely to be most fruitful. For the adult cancers, somatic regions of homozygous deletion analogous to the chromomsome 18q region, which contains the DCC gene, are likely to be present in many cases, and have actually been described in a number of instances. However, the clues that permit the direct identification of such regions are likely to be less straightforward than those for the childhood cancers for a number of reasons. The technological developments that embody the Human Genome Initiative should have a major bearing on this search. The identification and characterization of a well-catalogued and precisely mapped series of expressed genes within a chromosomal region suspected to harbor a tumor-suppressor gene will clearly facilitate the search for such genes. The prospects for the identification of the full range of tumor-suppressor genes using these newly developed metodologies and data bases are in my view, extraordinarily promising.

References

Buckler, A. J., Pelletier, J., Haber, D. A. *et al.* (1991). Isolation, characterization, and expression of the murine Wilms' tumor gene (WT1) during kidney development. *Mol. Cell. Biol.* **11**, 1701–1712.

Call, K. M., Glaser, T. M., Ito, C. Y. *et al.* (1990). Isolation and characterization of a zinc-finger polypeptide gene at the human chromosome 11 Wilms' tumor locus. *Cell* **60**, 509–520.

Crowell, J. K., Wadey, R. B., Haber, D. A., Call, K. M., Housman, D. E., and Prichard, D. J. (1991). Rearrangements of the WT1 gene in Wilms' tumor cell. *Oncogene* **6**, 595–599.

Dracopoli, N. C., Ahadeff, B., Houghton, A. N., and Old, L. J. (1987). Loss of heterozygosity at autosomal and X-linked loci during tumor progression in a patient with melanoma. *Cancer Res.* **47**, 3995.

Dryja, T. P., Rapaport, J. M., Joyce, J. M., and Peterson, R. A. (1986). Molecular detection of deletions involving band q14 of chromosome 13 in retinoblastomas. *Proc. Natl. Acad. Sci. U.S.A.* **83**, 7391.

Fearon, E. R., Cho, K., Nigro, J., Kern, J., Simons, S., Ruppert, J., *et al.* (1990). Identification of a chromosome 18q gene that is altered in colorectal cancers. *Science* **247**, 49–56.

Friend, S. H., Horowitz, J. M., Gerber, M. R. *et al.* (1987). Deletions of a DNA sequence in retinbolastomas and mesenchymal tumors: Organization of the sequence and its encoded protein. *Proc. Natl. Acad. Sci. U.S.A.* **84**, 9059–9063.

Gessler, M., Poustka, A., Cavenee, W. *et al.* (1990). Homozygous deletion in Wilms' tumours of a zinc-finger gene identified by chromosome jumping. *Nature (London)* **343**, 774–778.

Glaser, T., Lane, T., and Housman, D. (1990). A mouse model of the Aniridia-Wilms' tumor deletion syndrome. *Science* **250**, 823–827.

Grundy, P., Koufos, A., Morgan, K. *et al.* (1988). Familiar predisposition to Wilms' tumour does not map to the short arm of chromosome 11. *Nature (London)* **336**, 374–376.

Haber, D. A., Buckler, A. J., Glaser, K. M. *et al.* (1990). An internal deletion within an 11p13 zinc-finger gene contributes to the development of Wilms' tumor. *Cell* **61**, 1257–1269.

Haber, D. A., Sohn, R., Buckler, A. R., Pelletier, J., Call, K, and Housman, D. E. (1991). Alternative splicing and genomic structure of the Wilms' tumor gene, WT1. *PNAS.* USA (in press).

Harris, H., Miller, Q. J., Klein, G. *et al.* (1969). Suppression of malignancy by cell fusion. *Nature (London)* **223**, 363–368.

Huff, V., Compton, D. A., Chao, L. Y. *et al.* (1988). Lack of linkage of familial Wilms' tumor to chromosome 11p13 markers. *Am. J. Hum. Genet.* **43**, A25.

Huff, V., Miwa, H., Haber, D. *et al.* (1991). Evidence for WTI as a Wilms' tumor (WT) gene: Intragenic germinal deletion in bilateral WT. *Am. J. Hum. Genet.* **48**, 997–1003.

Knudson, A. G. (1971). Mutation and cancer: A statistical study. *Proc. Natl. Acad. Sci. U.S.A.* **68**, 820.

Knudson, A. G., and Strong, L. C. (1972). Mutation and cancer: A model for Wilms' tumor of the kidney. *J. Natl. Cancer Inst.* **48**, 313.

Koufos, A., Grundy, P., Morgan, K. *et al.* (1989). Familial Wiedemann-Beckwith syndrome and a second Wilms' tumor locus map to 11p15.5. *Am. J. Hum. Genet.* **44,** 711–719.

Lee, W. H., Bodestein, R., Hong, F. *et al.* (1987). Human retinoblastoma susceptibility gene: Cloning, identification, and sequence. *Science* **235,** 1394–1399.

Lewis, W. H., Yeger, H., Bonetta, L. *et al.*, (1988). Homozygous deletion of a DNA marker from chromosome 11p13 in sporadic Wilms' tumor. *Genomics* **3,** 25.

Mannens, M., Slater, R. M., Heyting, C. *et al.* (1987). Chromosome 11, Wilms' tumor and associated congenital diseases. *Cytogenet. Cell Genet.* **46,** 655.

Miller, R. W., Fraumeni, J. F., and Manning, M. D. (1964). Association of Wilms' tumor with aniridia, hemihypertrophy, and other congenital anomalies. *N. Engl. J. Med.* **270,** 922.

Mitchell, P. J., and Tijan, T. (1989). Transcriptional regulation in mammalian cells by sequence-specific DNA binding proteins. *Science* **245,** 371–378.

Pelletier, J., Shalling, M., Buckler, A. J., Rogers, A., Haber, D. A., and Housman, D. (1991). Expression of the Wilms' tumor gene WT1 in the murine urogenetital system. *Genes and Development* **5,** 1545–1556.

Pritchard-Jones, K., Fleming, S., Davidson, D. *et al.* (1990). The candidate Wilms' tumour gene is involved in genitourinary development. *Nature (London)* **346,** 194–197.

Reeve, A. E., Sih, S. A., Ralzis, A. M. *et al.* (1989). Loss of allelic heterozygosity at a second locus on chromosome 11 in Wilms' tumor cells. *Mol. Cell. Biol.* **9,** 1799–1803.

Rausher, F. J. III, Morris, J. F., Tournay, O. E. *et al.* (1990). Binding of the Wilms' tumor locus zinc-finger protein to the EGR1 consensus sequence. *Science* **250,** 1259–1262.

Riccardi, V. M., Sujansky, E., Smith, A. C. *et al.* (1978). Chromosomal imbalance in the aniridia–Wilms' tumor association: 11p interstitial deletion. *Pediatrics* **61,** 604.

Rose, E. A., Glaser, T. M., Jones, C. A. *et al.* (1990). Complete physical map of the WAGR region of 11p13 localizes a candidate Wilms' tumor gene. *Cell* **60,** 495–508.

Sager, R. (1985). Genetic suppression of tumor formation. *Adv. Cancer Res.* **44,** 43–68.

Schwartz, C., Haber, D., Stanton, V., Strong, L., Skolnick, M., and Housman, D. (1991). Familial predisposition to Wilms' tumor does not segregate with the WT1 gene. *Genomics* **10,** 927.

Sotelo-Avila, C. F., Gonzalez-Crossi, F., and Fowler, J. M. (1980). Complete and incomplete forms of Beckwith-Wiedemann syndrome: Their oncogenic potential. *J. Pediatr.* **96,** 47–50.

Ton, C., Hoff, V., Call, K. M. *et al.* (1991). Smallest region of overlap in Wilms' tumor deletions uniquely implicates an 11p13 zinc-finger gene as the disease locus. *Genomics* **10,** 293–297.

Waziri, M., Patil, S. E., Hanson, J. W., and Bartley, J. A. (1983). Abnormality of chromosome 11 in patients with features of Beckwith-Wiedemann syndrome. *J. Pediatr.* **102,** 873–876.

Yunis, J. J., and Ramsey, N. (1978). Retinoblastoma and subband deletion of chromosome 13. *Am. J. Dis. Child.* **132,** 161.

PART III

Regulation of Transcription

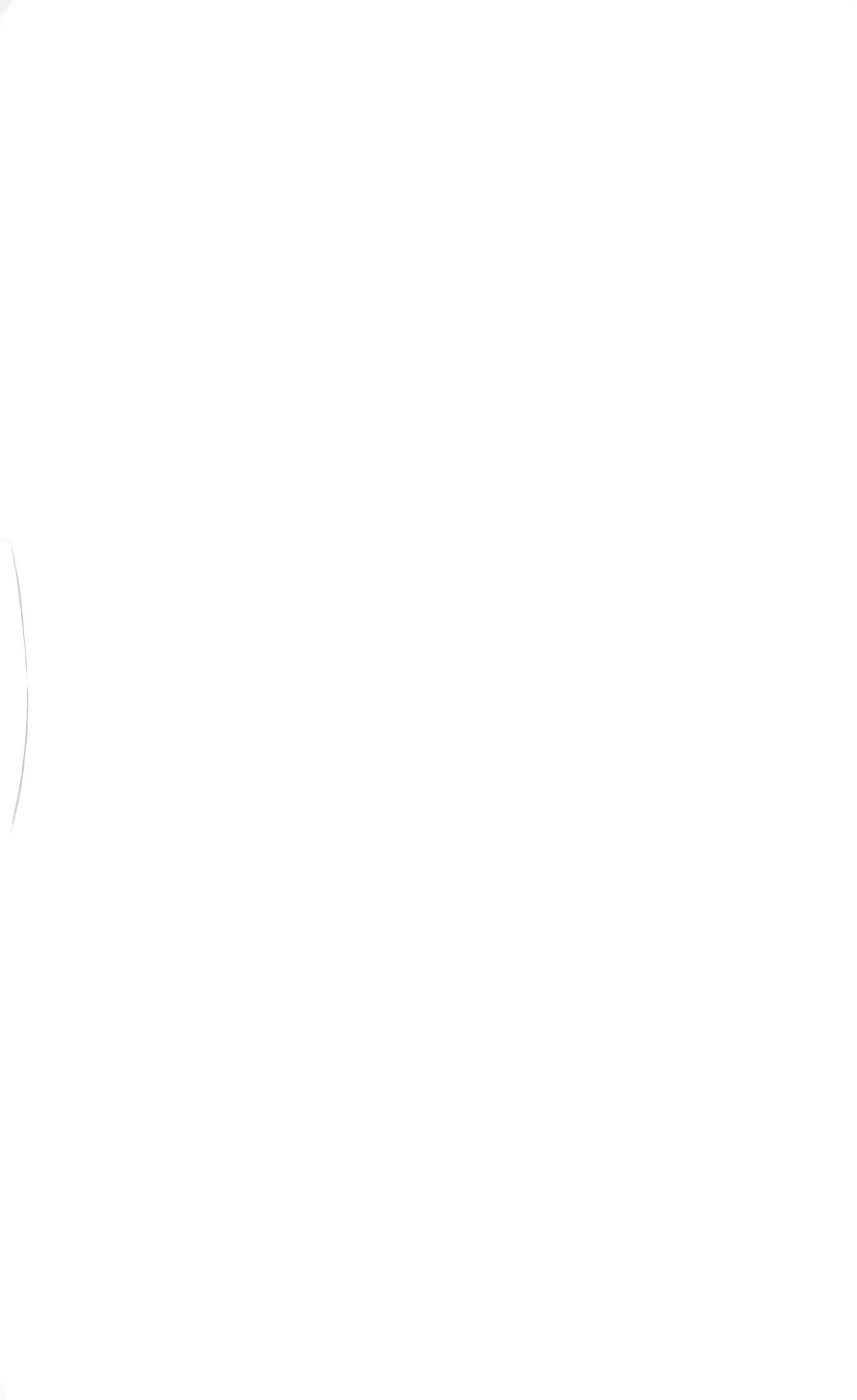

10

The Serum Response Element: Structure and Function

RICHARD TREISMAN

Transcription Laboratory
Imperial Cancer Research Fund
Lincoln's Inn Fields
London, United Kingdom

NUCLEAR PROCESSES
AND ONCOGENES

I. Introduction

Stimulation of cells by growth factors or mitogens transiently activates the transcription of a large family of genes, including the protooncogenes c-*fos*, c-*jun*, c-*myc* and c-*rel*, without the need for prior protein synthesis. Many of these cellular *immediate-early* genes encode transcriptional regulatory proteins, the expression of which in turn determines the subsequent response of the genome, and ultimately of the cell, to growth factor stimulation (see Bravo, 1990). Control of the signal-transduction process is of cardinal importance in the control of cell growth. For example, inhibition of c-*fos* gene expression during exposure of quiescent cells to serum prevents progress into S phase and subsequent mitosis (Nishikura and Murray, 1987; Holt *et al.*, 1986; Riabowol *et al.*, 1988). The elucidation of the molecular mechanism by which immediate-early gene expression is regulated will therefore be a major step toward understanding regulation of cell growth processes. This chapter examines the serum response element (SRE), an important immediate-early gene regulatory element, and considers in detail the structure and possible functions of one of its binding proteins, serum response factor (SRF).

II. The Serum Response Element

A common regulatory element, the serum response element (SRE; Treisman, 1985, 1986; Gilman *et al.*, 1986; Greenberg *et al.*, 1987), has been identified, which is in large part responsible for transcriptional regulation of the c-*fos* and several other cellular immediate-early genes. SRE sequences function to a large extent independent of their position and orientation relative to other promoter elements and the mRNA cap site; this is reflected in the wide variety of locations in which the SRE is found in different immediate-early gene promoters. The SRE acts as a basal promoter element, and its transcriptional activity is rapidly increased following stimulation of cell by many different growth factors. Activation of the SRE involves signal transduction by both protein kinase C-dependent and -independent mechanisms (see Rivera and Greenberg, 1990; Treisman, 1990); its activation is linked to signal pathways involving *ras* (Sassonne-Corsi *et al.*, 1989; Gauthier-Rouviere *et al.*, 1990), *raf* (Kaibuchi *et al.*, 1989; Jamal and Ziff, 1990; Siegfried and Ziff, 1990), and HTLV-I tax protein (Fujii *et al.*, 1989). The down-regulation of SRE activity is achieved at least in part by an autoregulatory mechanism that involves two immediate-early gene products, Fos and Jun (Sassonne Corsi *et al.*, 1988; Schontal *et al.*, 1989; Wilson and Treisman, 1988; Lucibello *et al.*, 1989; Konig *et al.*, 1989; Gius *et al.*, 1990). The mechanism of SRE function is thus of considerable interest from the points of view of both signal transduction and transcriptional regulation.

The sequence of the c-*fos* SRE is compared to other characterized SRE sequences in Fig. 1. The c-*fos* SRE contains a 20 basepair imperfect dyad symmetry, and the term DSE (for dyad symmetry element) has therefore also been used; however, as can be seen from Fig. 1, not all SREs contain dyad symmetries, and the discussion that follows will keep to the more descriptive term SRE. The prototype SRE was defined in the regulatory sequences of the human c-*fos* gene as the binding site for a ubiquitous nuclear protein termed serum response factor (SRF); cDNA clones encoding this protein have been isolated (Norman *et al.*, 1988). The SRE alone can mediate transient transcription induction with perfectly normal kinetics when excised from its normal position and linked to a heterologous promoter (Konig *et al.*, 1989), although a number of different proteins bind in its vicinity *in vivo* (Herrera *et al.*, 1989; Fig. 1). Furthermore, SREs from different immediate-early gene promoters share only the sequence $CC(A/T)_6GG$, embedded in contexts that usually lack significant dyad symmetry (Fig. 1). As will be described, this sequence represents the core SRF-binding site: SRE mutations that reduce or prevent SRF binding have parallel effects on the inducibility of the SRE by growth factors. A genomic footprinting study of the c-*fos* SRE in A431 cells showed that a footprint characteristic of SRF is present before, during, and after stimulation by epidermal growth factor (Herrera *et al.*, 1989).

The above data suggest that SRF plays a major role in signal transduction at the SRE; however, a number of observations suggest that this view may be an oversimplification. First, a number of other $CC(A/T)_6GG$ box-binding proteins have been identified in DNA binding assays and by molecular cloning: it is unlikely that SRF and these other factors can bind the SRE simultaneously. Second, SRF bound at the c-*fos* SRE forms a ternary complex with another protein, $p62^{TCF}$, which makes contacts with the DNA to the left of SRF (Fig. 1), and in some cases, mutations at these positions affect growth-factor activation of the SRE (Shaw *et al.*, 1989; Graham and Gilman, 1991). Third, $CC(A/T)_6GG$ boxes form essential elements of a number of muscle-specific promoters (Minty and Kedes, 1986; Miwa and Kedes, 1987; Muscat *et al.*, 1988; Walsh and Schimmel, 1988;

```
c-fos^H,M       A C A C A G G A T G T C C A T A.T T A G G A C A T C T G C G T C A

SRF                               x   X X           X X   x     x
SRF:p62/TCF               X X     X   X X           X X   x     x
A431 in vivo              X X     X   X X           X X   X     X   X X X   X

γ-actin^X       C T G A A A G A T G C C C A T A.T T T G G C G A T C T T C T G T C

krox20/2        C C G G A T C T T C T C C T T T.T T T G G A A A G T C T C G G A G

krox20/1        T G T T C C T C A G T C C A T A.T A T G G G C A G C G A C G T C A

zif268/1        C T T C C T G C T T C C C A T A.T A T G G C C A T G T A C G T C A

zif268/2        G G T C G G T C C T T C C A T A.T T A G G G C T T C C T G C T T C

zif268/3        T T T C C C C A G C G C C T T A.T A T G G A G T G G C C C A A T A
```

```
zif268/4          A C C C G G A A A C G C C A T A.T A A G G A G C A G G A A G G A T
β-actinH/TATA     T C C G A A A G T T G C C T T T.T A T G G C T C G A G C G G C C G
β-actinH/IVS1     A C C A G T G T T T G C C T T T.T A T G G T A A T A A C G C G G C

CONSENSUS                   _ _ A T(A A)C C A T A.T A T G G(T T)A T _ _
                                C           T   T   T A           G
```

Fig. 1. The c-*fos* and other immediate-early gene SRE sequences. The sequence of the human/mouse c-*fos* SRE is shown at the top; crosses indicate the positions of the top strand DMS footprints for *in vitro* binding of the SRF and SRF:p62TCF complexes, and the genomic footprint observed in A431 cells *in vivo* (data from Herrara *et al.*, 1989). The sequences of ten proven SRE sequences are shown, with a derived consensus below. Underlined regions indicate oligonucleotide regions derived from these sequences that retain full SRE activity, except for the two human actin SREs, where they indicate locations of mutations that block SRE function. Overlined regions indicate an AP1/ATF-like present at the same location relative to three of the SREs.

Mohun *et al.*, 1989; Chow and Schwartz, 1990), which can also bind SRF (Boxer *et al.*, 1989; Taylor *et al.*, 1989; Gustafson *et al.*, 1989). These muscle gene $CC(A/T)_6GG$ boxes exhibit preferential activity in muscle cells, but can function as effective SREs in nonmuscle cells (Walsh, 1989; Taylor *et al.*, 1989; Tuil *et al.*, 1990).

III. Serum Response Element-Binding Proteins

A number of SRE-binding proteins have been identified, using the sensitive band-shift or DNA affinity precipitation (DNAP) assays, and three have been characterized in some detail. It is possible that other SRE-binding proteins remain undetected, since the results obtained with these assays are very dependent on the particular methods used. This section reviews the properties of three proteins: serum response factor (SRF; Treisman, 1986; Gilman *et al.*, 1986; Prywes and Roeder, 1986; Greenberg *et al.*, 1987), p62 (Walsh and Schimmel, 1987; Ryan *et al.*, 1989), and $p62^{TCF}$ (ternary complex factor; Shaw *et al.*, 1989a).

A. Serum Response Factor

Serum response factor (SRF) is a ubiquitous nuclear polypeptide of apparent M_r 62–67 kDa defined by sodium dodecyl sulfate-polyacrylamide gel electrophoresis (SDS-PAGE) (Treisman, 1987; Prywes and Roeder, 1987; Schroter *et al.*, 1987; Ryan *et al.*, 1989). The protein is phosphorylated on serines *in vivo* (Prywes *et al.*, 1988; Manak *et al.*, 1990; Schalasta and Doppler, 1990) and contains O-linked *N*-acetylglucosamine (Schroter *et al.*, 1990). SRF cDNA clones encode a polypeptide of predicted M_r 51,093, rich in serine and threonine, which contains potential recognition sites for casein kinase II (CK II) and protein kinase A (Norman *et al.*, 1988). The SRF gene is highly conserved between species, and its mRNAs are themselves inducible by serum stimulation in HeLa cells. In an *in vitro* transcription assay, SRF functions as a constitutive transcriptional activator (Norman *et al.*, 1988; Manak *et al.*, 1990), and expression of a LexA-SRF fusion gene in 3T3 cells is sufficient to render a LexA operator weakly serum inducible (S. John and R. Treisman, manuscript in preparation). Two yeast regulatory proteins, MCM1 and ARG80, contain regions highly homologous (70% identity) to the SRF DNA-binding domain (Dubois *et al.*, 1987; Norman *et al.*, 1988; Passmore *et al.*, 1988; Ammerer, 1989).

In most extracts obtained from cell lines and tissues, SRF is readily detectable by band-shift or DNAP assay, and binding activity does not appear to change after growth factor stimulation (Treisman, 1986; Greenberg *et al.*, 1987; Prywes and Roeder, 1986; Gilman *et al.*, 1986). In A431 cells, however, a substantial increase in SRE-binding activity after EGF treatment has been reported (Prywes and Roeder, 1986; Prywes *et al.*, 1988), but this is not reflected in changes in the c-*fos* SRE genomic footprint (Herrara *et al.*, 1989). *In vitro* studies show that SRF is indeed a substrate for CK II (Manak *et al.*, 1990; Marais *et al.*, 1992), and that phosphorylation by this enzyme acts to potentiate SRF-DNA exchange rates rather than modulate binding affinity (Marais *et al.*, 1992). However, although CK II activity in several cell types increases upon growth factor stimulation (Sommercorn *et al.*, 1987), it remains to be proven directly that CKII phosphorylation regulates SRF activity *in vivo*. The means by which this phosphorylation regulates SRF-DNA binding is unknown: it would appear unlikely that phosphorylation alters a conserved structure so as to cause an allosteric change in the DNA-binding domain, because the context of the N-terminal CK II site is totally divergent between human and xenopus SRF (Mohun *et al.*, 1991). Although phosphorylation is not necessary for binding *per se:* SRF expressed in bacteria, or that lacks the CK II site, exhibits readily detectable specific DNA-binding activity (Norman *et al.*, 1988; Manak *et al.*, 1990). However, treatment of SRF in crude extracts with phosphatase causes virtually complete loss of DNA-binding activity (Prywes *et al.*, 1988a; Boxer *et al.*, 1988; Schalasta and Doppler, 1989); perhaps an additional factor present in crude cell extracts blocks SRE binding by dephosphorylated SRF, or dephosphorylation may activate an inhibitory factor. Further studies are necessary to resolve this issue.

B. Ternary Complex Factor

The ternary complex factor (p62^{TCF}) protein was initially identified as an activity that in band-shift assays caused further retardation of the SRF:SRE complex; biochemical studies identified this as a ~62 kDa polypeptide(s), with no apparent specific affinity for SRE DNA in the absence of SRF (Shaw *et al.*, 1989a). The protein is not glycosylated, and binds to an SRF dimer, increasing its apparent affinity for the SRE some 50-fold (Schroter *et al.*, 1990). Studies using truncated derivatives of SRF indicate that $p62^{TCF}$ interaction occurs via the SRF DNA-binding domain itself rather than other parts of the molecule (Schroter *et al.*, 1990; R. T., unpublished data).

Methylation interference analysis of the interaction at the c-*fos* SRE identified two G contacts unique to the $p62^{TCF}$:SRF:SRE complex at positions −10 and −11 (Fig. 1); a transversion mutation that changes this sequence from ACAGG to AACTG blocks binding of $p62^{TCF}$ to the SRF:SRE complex. Position −9 of the c-*fos* SRE has also been implicated in $p62^{TCF}$ contact in a mutational study of ternary complex formation (Graham and Gilman, 1991). *In vivo* footprinting of the c-*fos* SRE in A431 cells shows binding of a $p62^{TCF}$-like protein before, during, and after stimulation with EGF (Herrera *et al.*, 1989). The $p62^{TCF}$ contacts are not generally conserved among known SREs, even between the c-*fos* SRE of different species such as frog and chicken (see Fig. 1). Perhaps sequence changes in the SRF-binding site can compensate for nonoptimal contacts between $p62^{TCF}$ and DNA; alternatively, it is possible that the ability to recruit $p62^{TCF}$ is not a property of all SREs. It will be interesting to investigate further the sequence specificity of $p62^{TCF}$:SRE interaction.

C. p62

This SRE-binding phosphoprotein, distinct from $p62^{TCF}$, was initially identified in H9 cells by the DNAP assay, and is abundant in many cell types. The chromatographic and DNA-binding properties of p62 suggest that it is probably the same factor as another previously identified $CC(A/T)_6GG$ box-binding protein, MAPF1 (Walsh and Schimmel, 1987). Analysis by DNAP assay and one-dimensional gel electrophoresis revealed that no obvious changes in labeling of the protein occur after growth factor stimulation (Ryan *et al.*, 1989). Methylation interference experiments using the c-*fos* SRE show that p62 contacts the CG base pairs at dyad positions −4 and −5 and makes additional close contacts at positions −7 and −10, suggesting that the protein binds at the left side of the dyad. The shared contact points of p62 and SRF make it unlikely that these proteins can simultaneously occupy the SRE.

D. Other SRE-Binding Proteins

Two other SRE-binding activities have been reported, although not characterized in detail. One of these, MAPF2 (Walsh and Schimmel, 1987), gives an identical methylation interference pattern to that of p62 (Ryan *et al.*, 1989), and is of M_r 35 kDa, defined by gel filtration. MAPF2 is found in many cell types (Walsh and Schimmel, 1987; Walsh, 1989). Another activity is detectable in extracts from neonatal murine tissues and has been denoted band I; binding studies indicate that this protein contacts the c-*fos* SRE at position +10, and also requires base pairs in the dyad center and right side (Levi *et al.*, 1989).

IV. Interaction of the Serum Response Factor with DNA

A. The SRF DNA-Binding Domain

SRF binds to DNA as a dimer, with an apparent K_d of 0.5 to 3 × 10^{11}M (Prywes and Roeder, 1987; Schroter *et al.*, 1990), similar to other eukaryotic sequence-specific DNA binding proteins, and some 10^5-fold greater than its affinity for nonspecific DNA (Prywes and Roeder, 1987). The protein makes close contacts with DNA at the CC and GG base pairs of the core sequence $CC(A/T)_6GG$, one DNA helical turn apart (Treisman, 1986; Gilman *et al.*, 1986; Prywes and Roeder, 1986; Greenberg *et al.*, 1987), and it is reasonable to assume that these reflect individual contacts by the two subunits. Experiments in which an SRF-binding site is located at different positions along a DNA fragment suggest SRF binding bends the DNA (Gustafson *et al.*, 1989).

The SRF DNA-binding domain was mapped using deletion derivatives of the protein produced by cell-free translation and corresponds to the region of 70% homology to the *Saccharomyces cerevisiae* MCM1 and ARG80 proteins, which recognize SRE-like sequences (Norman *et al.*, 1988; Hayes *et al.*, 1988; Passmore *et al.*, 1989; Ammerer, 1989). However, inclusion of some forty amino acids C-terminal to the homology region is required for high-affinity binding (Norman *et al.*, 1988). The DNA-binding domain also includes sequences required for dimerization, and the two functions are to some extent separable; deletions within its highly basic N-terminal region block DNA binding but allow dimerization. However, the C-terminal border of the DNA-binding domain coincides with the C-terminal border of the dimerization region. The basic region is therefore likely to be directly involved in sequence-specific DNA recognition. The SRF DNA-binding domain contains no sequence motifs previously associated with sequence-specific DNA binding; structural predictions suggest that the N-terminal basic region probably comprises two helical segments separated by regions of turn and β sheet. The N-terminal half of the dimerization region is rich in hydrophobic residues.

A number of other proteins share homology to the SRF DNA-binding domain (Sommer *et al.*, 1990; Yanofsky *et al.*, 1990; Pollock and Treisman, 1991). All of these proteins exhibit striking homology with the N-terminal basic region and the hydrophobic segment of the dimerization region; however at least two of them recognize different binding sites from those recognized by SRF (Pollock and Treisman, 1991). A simple view of the high degree of sequence conservation between SRF-like DNA-binding domains is thus that the basic regions contain a common structural framework upon which sequence-specific features are displayed. Ultimately, it may be possible to discern a recognition code associating particular amino acids in the DNA-binding domain with specific-sequence features. It remains possible, however, that the different dimerization regions also play an indirect role in determination of sequence specificity by changing the relative position of the conserved basic region with respect to the DNA.

B. DNA-Binding Specificity of SRF

1. *Mutagenesis Studies*

The sequence specificity of SRF:DNA interaction has been studied using mutant SREs, principally derived from the c-*fos* SRE. These studies suggested that three considerations affect the affinity of SRF for the SRE: (1) presence of the close CC and GG contact points at positions +/−4 and +/−5 relative to the dyad; (2) the integrity and sequence of the A/T-rich core sequence; (3) the sequences flanking the core $CC(A/T)_6GG$ box. Some but not all totally symmetrized sites exhibit very high apparent affinity for SRF (Treisman, 1987), and it has been suggested that the symmetric elements of the c-*fos* SRE act to increase binding affinity (Rivera *et al.*, 1990); however, subsequent studies have shown that affinity of symmetrized sites may result from the binding conditions used (Ryan *et al.*, 1989).

Methylation interference studies suggest that SRF makes close contacts with the DNA at the G-C basepairs at positions +/−4 and +/−5 relative to the dyad (Treisman, 1986; Gilman *et al.,* 1986; Prywes and Roeder, 1986; Greenberg *et al.,* 1987). Symmetrically placed mutations at these positions, or deletions encompassing them, block binding entirely (Treisman, 1987; Greenberg *et al.,* 1987; Gilman, 1988). In the c-*fos* SRE, single mutations at these positions reduce binding affinity more than 10-fold, but do not necessarily block binding (Leung and Miyamoto, 1989). Deletion of an AT base pair from the A/T-rich sequence of the CC(A/T)$_6$GG box in the center of SREs blocks SRF binding (Christy and Nathans, 1989; Subramanian *et al.,* 1989; Phan-Dinh-Tuy *et al.,* 1989), whereas mutations that introduce C or G residues reduce affinity (Leung and Miyamoto, 1989). Binding affinity is apparently partly determined by the sequence of AT basepairs; changes in the sequence of the central AT region of the c-*fos* SRE can substantially affect binding affinity (Leung and Miyamoto, 1989). Several studies confirm that the context of a CC(A/T)$_6$GG box affects SRF-binding affinity. First, methylation of base pairs outside the CC(A/T)$_6$GG can interfere with SRF binding (Mohun *et al.,* 1987). Second, placement of identical CC(A/T)$_6$GG core sequences in different sequence contexts, or mutations of the flanking sequences in the Fos SRE, give binding sites of different affinities (Norman and Treisman, 1988; Shaw *et al.,* 1989a; Rivera *et al.,* 1990; Fredrickson *et al.,* 1989; Leung and Miyamoto, 1989).

2. Selection of SRF-Binding Sites de Novo

We used a novel technique to study the binding specificity of SRF in which the protein is used to select high-affinity binding sites from a pool of random sequence oligonucleotides (Pollock and Treisman, 1990). Our strategy, based on the indirect immunoprecipitation of DNA, is shown in Fig. 2. Protein is allowed to interact with a pool of radiolabeled oligonucleotides, which consist of a central random sequence flanked by two primer sequences for the polymerase chain reaction (PCR). Complexes are recovered by immunoprecipitation, and subjected to a gentle wash; DNA recovery is monitored by scintillation counting. The bound DNA is then eluted and amplified using the PCR. The amplified DNA is then used for another round of binding selection and amplification, or used in a DNA-binding assay with the selecting protein. The immunopurification method does not require the overproduction and purification of the protein concerned;

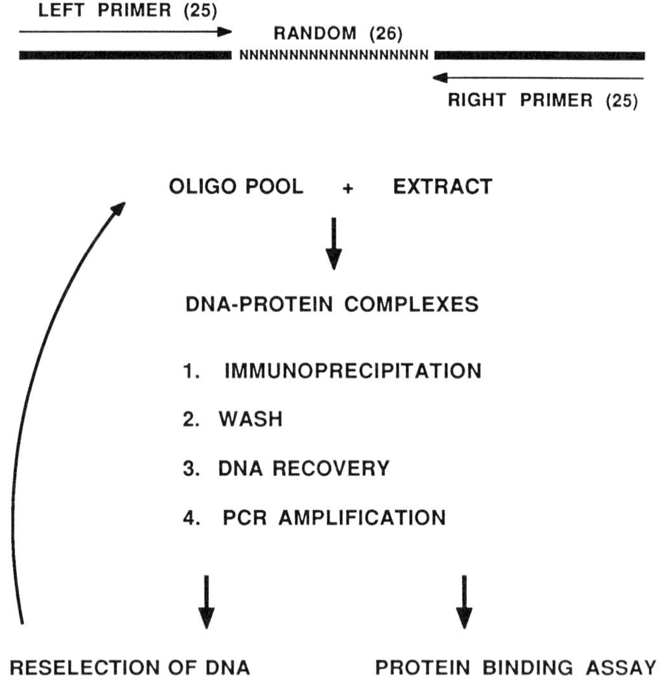

Fig. 2. Binding-site selection protocol. Top, the oligonucleotides used: a 26-base completely random sequence is flanked by two 25-base PCR primer sequences that contain restriction sites to allow cloning of selected DNA. Below, the steps in selection of binding sites from the random oligonucleotide pool. Oligonucleotide amplification is performed using radiolabel so as to facilitate quantitation and analysis by DNA-binding assay.

since binding reactions can be performed using protein present in nuclear extracts or cell-free translations, the method can be used with proteins that bind as heterodimers or that require posttranslational modifications in order to bind DNA. Selections are performed under conditions in which the selecting protein is initially in substantial molar excess over binding sites in the oligonucleotide pool, so initial selection will be for sites that bind above an affinity threshold effectively defined by the concentration of selecting protein and the binding and wash conditions. In later rounds of selection, the proportion of molecules in the population that carry binding sites will increase to a point at which the selecting protein is no longer in excess, and selection of higher affinity sites will occur.

We evaluated the DNA-binding specificity of SRF produced by *in vitro* translation. Progress of the procedure was monitored by measuring the percentage of input probe recovered for each selection cycle, and by testing the selected DNA in gel mobility-shift assays. As the binding-site selection proceeds, the probe oligonucleotide pools should become enriched in sequences that can bind SRF, and consistent with this, increasing proportions of input DNA were recovered on successive rounds of selection. In the gel mobility-shift assay, this selected DNA forms complexes containing SRF as judged by their reactivity with the selecting SRF antibody. To examine the general character of the selected DNA, we performed binding-competition studies. We tested whether the selected sites were of the $CC(A/T)_6GG$ type by including in the binding reactions increasing amounts of either an unlabeled wild-type *c-fos* SRE oligonucleotide or a non-binding mutant oligonucleotide that carries C → G transversions at position −/+4 relative to the dyad. This analysis confirmed that the vast majority of the selected sites must be of the type found in the *c-fos* SRE; in addition, direct binding analyses of twelve cloned sites confirmed that the sites were of affinity comparable to that of the *c-fos* SRE.

3. *Characteristics of High-Affinity SRF-Binding Sites*

The DNA recovered after two rounds of selection was purified, cloned, and analyzed by DNA sequencing; results are shown in Fig. 3. The half site consensus, 5′ A/C-A/T-G/T-A/C-C-C-A/T-T/A-A 3′, matches the previously deduced SRF-binding site consensus well. All but one of the sites present after two rounds of selection contained the invariant CC and GG contact points, and no sites containing GC basepairs in the central region were recovered. Certain patterns of AT base pairs in the central region were preferred: only a subset of the possible patterns of the six A/T residues at the core of the site was recovered. The central A/T dinucleotide appears invariant, as expected from the large number of naturally occurring sites of this type, and few sites contained five or more adenosines out of six.

This analysis of the selected sequences shows that although SRF recognizes an essentially dyad symmetrical DNA operator, its interactions with each half of the dyad are not absolutely equivalent: a striking example of this is seen at positions +/−6: +6, T; −6, C (Fig. 3). Since SRF bends DNA upon binding, this may reflect selection for an asymmetry in the location of the center of DNA bending under our

```
S2 10      gaattcgcctcCACGGGCATTCCATATATAGTAACATcgacaggatcc

S2         ggatcctgtcgTTTCGAACCACATATGACCATATATGGaggcgaattc
S2 12      ggatcctgtcgAACTGACCATATATGGAAGTAACTTTgaggcgaattc
S2 14      ggatcctgtcgGTCTAATGACCATATATGGGTAATACgaggcgaattc
S2 19      gaattcgcctcATGCCCATATATGGTCCGTAGATAAAcgacaggatcc
S2 21      gaattcgcctcGTGCCCATATATGGTGTTAATGACAGcgacaggatcc
S2 26      gaattcgcctcAAGATCATGCCCATATATGGTAGTTCcgacaggatcc
S2 27      gaattcgcctcAATGTCCATATATGGTATTGTCTTACcgacaggatcc
S2 29      gaattcgcctcTAAAACAGTCCGAGCCATATATGGTGcgacaggatcc
S2 30      ggatcctgtcgATGACCATATATGGCATTTGCACTATgaggcgaattc
S2 3.3     gaattcgcctcCGGGACATGTCCATATATGGAGTGTAcgacaggatcc
S2 5.3     gaattcgcctcACTGCCCATATATGGCGTTGTACGTCcgacaggatcc
S2 29.3    gaattcgcctcACCGCCCATATATGGTTATGTGCCTTcgacaggatcc
S2 5.2     ggatcctgtcgGACCTTTATGCCCATATATGGCATT gaggcgaattc
S2 17.2    gaattcgcctcCATATATGGATAATACATAGGCTAATcgacaggatcc
S2 18.2    ggatcctgtcgAGTTGACACAATACCATATATGGTATgaggcgaattc
S2 22.2    ggatcctgtcgAAGCTTATGCCCATATATGGGTATGCgaggcgaattc

S2 23      gaattcgcctcATAAAACGTAATATGTCCATATAAGGcgacaggatcc
S2 12.3    gaattcgcctcTTGTGCCCATATAAGGTAATGGTTAGcgacaggatcc
S2 29.2    ggatcctgtcgGATACATGACCATATAAGGGCCATAGgaggcgaattc
S2 ·11     ggatcctgtcgCTTATGCCCATATAAGGTTCTAAGGgaggcgaattc
S2 1       ggatcctgtcgCAGCAATGCCCATATAAGGCAATATgaggcgaattc
S2 2       ggatcctgtcgTTGTTACCATGCCCTTATATGGAGCCgaggcgaattc
S2 8       ggatcctgtcgGTAGATCATGCCCTTATATGGAAACAgaggcgaattc
S2 17      ggatcctgtcgTGCGGGTATTGCCCTTATATGGTCATgaggcgaattc
S2 25      ggatcctgtcgCATCCGGAAATTGTTGCCCTTATATGgaggcgaattc
S2 28      ggatcctgtcg TAGCGCAACATTAGTTCCTTATATGgaggcgaattc
S2 4       gaattcgcctcCTCTTAAATTACCTTATATGGTGTTAcgacaggatcc
S2 5       gaattcgcctcGGGCTATTACCTTATATGGTAGTCTTcgacaggatcc
S2 14.3    gaattcgcctcAAAGGACTTCCTTATATGGCACGTTGcgacaggatcc
S2 14.2    ggatcctgtcgAATGCCCTTATATGGGCGTCGCACA gaggcgaattc
S2 28.2    ggatcctgtcgTGCTCCATGCCCTTATATGGTACTGGgaggcgaattc

S2 18      ggatcctgtcgACGGTCTGATCACCTTATAAGGTAAGgaggcgaattc
S2 22      ggatcctgtcgAACAAAAGCCTTATAAGGCGTGCTAgaggcgaattc
S2 17.3    gaattcgcctcTTAATTACCTTATAAGGCTGTATGATcgacaggatcc
S2 19.3    ggatcctgtcgGAACCATTGCCCTTATAAGGATCGCCgaggcgaattc

S2 28      gaattcgcctcCTCGCCTATGCCCATATTTGGACGTCcgacaggatcc
S2 18.3    ggatcctgtcgTGCCCATATTTGGACATATAACTACAgaggcgaattc

S2 3.2     ggatcctgtcACGTATGCCCATATTAGGGTGGCAAA gaggcgaattc
S2 7       gaattcgcctcTAGATAGTTATGCCCATATTAGGAAGcgacaggatcc
S2 22.3    gaattcgcctcCTCTCACATGCCCATATTAGGAGCGTcgacaggatcc
S2 19.2    ggatcctgtcgCAAAGACAATGCCCATATTAGGCATTgaggcgaattc

S2 6.2     ggatcctgtcgGTCTTTATGCCCAAATTTGGGCCTTCgaggcgaattc

S2 3       gaattcgcctcGACCATTAACATGCCCAAATAAGGAGcgacaggatcc
S2 13      ggatcctgtcgGGGGTAATCATGCCCAAATAAGGTATGgaggcgaattc
```

CONSENSUS

A	27	2	1	8	-	-	23	2	35	-	30	12	1	-	7	15	9	2
G	2	-	28	1	-	-	-	-	-	-	-	-	34	35	6	7	7	9
C	4	2	1	22	35	35	-	-	-	-	-	-	-	-	8	6	9	3
T	2	31	5	4	-	-	12	23	-	35	5	23	-	-	14	7	10	21

HALF SITE

A	48	12	8	22	-	-	46	7	70
G	5	9	34	9	-	-	-	-	-
C	13	9	8	28	70	69	-	-	-
T	4	40	20	11	-	1	24	63	-

binding conditions, although we cannot exclude the possibility that asymmetric sites are selected by the PCR. Two other SRF-related proteins, the yeast MCM1 and mammalian RSRF.C4 proteins, also interact with their sites partially asymmetrically (Passmore *et al.*, 1989; RP and RT, manuscript in preparation).

Taken together, the results of this analysis show that the naturally occurring SRE sequences are very similar to SRF sites selected *in vitro*. However, some differences are apparent. For example, SRF binding *in vitro* is not favored by GC basepairs at position −/+6 (Fig. 3), whereas many SREs contain GC basepairs at these positions (Fig. 1). This may reflect the fact that protein-binding sites in genomic DNA may evolved to bind multiple proteins, or to exclude particular proteins: perhaps these sequences favor p62 binding to the SRE.

V. Mutational Analysis of the Serum Response Element

Considerable mutational analysis of the SRE has been performed in attempts to correlate binding of specific proteins with SRE function. Many studies have investigated SRE function in the context of the c-*fos* promoter, and these experiments must be interpreted carefully for two reasons. First, mutations will not necessarily specifically block access of only one protein to the SRE. Second, mutations that block protein binding to an SRE may allow proteins to bind to neighboring sites such as an AP1 site next to the c-*fos* SRE; their effects on transcription may result therefore be indirect (Shaw *et al.*, 1989b). Taken together, the data suggest that binding of SRF (or a protein with very similar sequence specificity) is required for inducibility of the SRE, but leave unclear the roles of other protein factors such as p62/MAPF1.

Mutations that block SRF binding, generally by changes of the

Fig. 3. Sequences of SRF-binding sites selected *de novo* from random-sequence DNA. The sites are aligned by the central CC(A/T)$_6$GG region present in each selected oligonucleotide, and grouped according to the type of A/T region present. The consensus sequences shown below were generated as follows (1) a half-site consensus was derived using all sequences; (2) all sequences where the half-site consensus overlaps the primer sequence were deleted from the data base; (3) a new half-site consensus was derived, and the sequences aligned so that the maximum half-site match is at the left.

central CC and GG SRF contact points, prevent the SRE-dependent induction of transcription by many different growth factors in diverse cell types (see Treisman, 1990, for review). In addition, in many cases mutations that reduce but do not block SRF binding have parallel effects on SRE inducibility (Treisman, 1987; Rivera *et al.*, 1990). It is likely that these mutations act by blocking the binding of SRF rather than the binding of other proteins such as p62/MAPF1 for the following reasons: first, inducibility is blocked by mutations that prevent SRF binding to the SRE but that would leave p62 binding intact (deletions of positions +4, +4 to +7; Greenberg *et al.*, 1987); second, p62/MAPF1 is not bound efficiently by a symmetrized synthetic derivative of the xenopus γ actin SRE that does function efficiently as an SRE (Treisman, 1987; Ryan *et al.*, 1989); third, the SRE is defined by the SRF-binding site core sequence $CC(A/T)_6GG$, rather than by the p62 binding site. The basal activity of the SRE and $CC(A/T)_6GG$ box is also dependent on both sets of SRF close contact points: transversions at positions +4 or −4 of both SREs and $CC(A/T)_6GG$ boxes from muscle-specific promoters block constitutive activity in both muscle and nonmuscle cells (Treisman, 1987; Walsh, 1989; Tuil *et al.*, 1990).

The role of the SRF:p62^{TCF} interaction in SRE function has been studied by testing the properties of mutant SREs, which cannot bind p62^{TCF}: in the case of the c-*fos*^{H} SRE, the results suggest that this interaction is important for regulated transcription. In one study, a nonbinding mutant exhibited a fourfold reduction in serum inducibility (Shaw *et al.*, 1989a); by contrast, another study showed that mutations of this type did not affect the response to serum factors, but reduced by 5- to 10-fold the response of the SRE to protein kinase C activators (Graham and Gilman, 1991). Other studies of c-*fos* SRE flanking sequence mutants, and of other SREs that lack p62^{TCF} contact points, found no differences in serum or phorbol ester inducibility compared to the intact c-*fos* SRE, although these studies did not evaluate p62^{TCF} binding directly (Rivera and Greenberg, 1990; Christy and Nathans, 1989). These apparent conflicts may arise from the differential dependence of serum activation on protein kinase C in different cell types, but it is clear that more needs to be done to evaluate the contribution of p62^{TCF} to activation of different SREs by different stimuli. A detailed analysis of the role of p62^{TCF} awaits the isolation of its cDNA.

Analysis of the sequence requirements for negative control of the c-*fos* and other immediate-early genes by Fos and Jun showed that this is a property of the SRE sequences in these promoters (Konig *et al.*, 1989; Gius *et al.*, 1990; Lucibello *et al.*, 1989). Both Fos-mediated and cycloheximide-sensitive negative regulation of the SRE require protein(s) with the sequence specificity of SRF; symmetric mutation of the SRF contact points, or a single base deletion in the A/T-rich center, blocks both serum and cycloheximide inducibility (Subramanian *et al.*, 1989; Gius *et al.*, 1990).

VI. The Role of the Serum Response Factor in Transcriptional Regulation

A. Growth Factor-Regulated Transcription

We have seen that the binding specificity of SRF defines an SRE, that SRF can recruit the $p62^{TCF}$ protein to the SRE, and that it contains a transactivation domain. In at least one situation, genomic footprinting indicates that proteins of specificity similar to those of the SRF:$p62^{TCF}$ complex are bound at the c-*fos* SRE before and during growth-factor stimulation. A simple model for SRE function is that SRF remains bound to the SRE throughout the induction process, and that its activity is modulated either by posttranslational modifications of SRF or proteins with which it interacts, or by accessory proteins that it recruits to the SRE. This *recruitment model* has the obvious attraction of analogy to the function of the *S. cerevisiae* MCM1 protein, whose activity is determined by accessory proteins, which it recruits in an operator-specific manner (reviewed by Herskowitz, 1989). However, it should be emphasized that it is not proven that MCM1 is a true SRF homolog.

According to the recruitment model, the activity of a particular SRF-binding site with respect to different signaling pathways could be modulated in three ways. First, the sequence context of a $CC(A/T)_6GG$ box could affect the ability of SRF to recruit accessory factors required for transduction of particular signals, a mechanism suggested to explain the differential response of mutants of the c-*fos* SRE defective in $p62^{TCF}$ binding to serum factors and PKC activators (Graham and Gilman, 1991). Second, the availability of particular accessory factors could vary according to cell type. Third, it is possible that the conformation of SRF itself depends on the primary sequence of its binding site; this might affect either its ability to recruit accessory proteins or its interaction with other components of the transcription apparatus, as proposed for the yeast MCM1 protein (Tan and Richmond, 1990). The basal level of SRE activity would be affected by these considerations and the relation of the SRE to other protein-binding sites in the promoter. Since at least in some cases it appears that protein binding to the SRE remains unchanged during stimulation, activation of the SRE would occur by modifications either of components of the complex or parts of the transcription machinery with which it interacts. Activation of the SRE in other situations could also involve regulation of accessory factor recruitment or of SRF DNA-binding activity. According to this view, the negative regulation of the SRE by Fos/Jun might occur indirectly via their interaction with SRF: such interactions have not been seen in gel mobility-shift assays (Gius *et al.,* 1990; Rivera *et al.,* 1990), but might be too weak to be detectable by this means.

An alternative model is that the protein complex at the SRE undergoes protein exchange during the induction process. If such exchanges were sufficiently rapid, they would not be detectable in genomic footprinting analysis, especially if they involved proteins of similar specificity to those bound before stimulation. A number of variants of this view are conceivable. For example SRF (and $p62^{TCF}$) might regulate basal transcription levels and, after growth factor stimulation, be replaced by a different, activated, complex; Fos and Jun would then act either to down-regulate the active complex, or generate a form of SRF that could replace it. This kind of model would provide potential roles for other $CC(A/T)_6GG$ box-binding proteins, such as p62/MAPF1, or proteins with similar DNA-binding specificities to SRF, although as yet the latter have not been detected.

Neither of these models provides a rationale for why SRF is itself an immediate-early gene. One possibility is that SRF is somehow inactivated or destroyed upon induction, and that newly synthesized protein is required to suppress SRE activity. Alternatively, fresh synthesis of SRF may increase levels of binding activity to allow binding at lower affinity sites inaccessible before stimulation, although this seems unlikely, since overall levels of binding activity appear relatively constant. The functional roles played by the regulation of SRF-binding activity and protein synthesis remain to be elucidated.

B. Muscle-Specific Transcription

The observation that apparently similar promoter elements are involved in activity both growth-factor responsive and muscle specific was unexpected and remains poorly understood. Three questions follow from this: (1) Do the same proteins, particularly SRF, participate in both muscle and nonmuscle $CC(A/T)_6GG$ box activity? (2) What determines the muscle-restricted activity of the muscle-specific $CC(A/T)_6GG$ boxes? (3) Are $CC(A/T)_6GG$ boxes always growth-factor responsive? At present the answers to these questions are not clear. A simple model is that SRF mediates $CC(A/T)_6GG$ box activity in both cell types. Consistent with this, muscle-specific $CC(A/T)_6GG$ box activity depends on both sets of SRF close contact points (Walsh, 1989), and muscle cells contain SRF (Boxer *et al.*, 1989; Taylor *et al.*, 1989). An alternative view is that different factors or combinations of factors with similar sequence specifities bind the muscle-specific $CC(A/T)_6GG$ boxes in the two situations. In this case the behavior of muscle-specific $CC(A/T)_6GG$ boxes in different cell types would be determined by relative abundance of the different factors, and their relative affinities for the site. The question as to whether the $CC(A/T)_6GG$ boxes found in muscle-specific promoters also act as SREs in muscle cells remains unanswered.

VII. Prospects

The SRF-binding site plays a crucial role in both growth factor-regulated and muscle-specific gene expression. Future work must concentrate on defining the functions of both SRF and the other various proteins that can interact with this site in growth factor-regulated and muscle-specific promoters. The availability of cDNAs encoding SRF should allow the development of systems to test directly its ability to regulate transcription in both nonmuscle and muscle cells, and to investigate its interactions with other proteins. The relationship of proteins such as $p62^{TCF}$ to regulation is intriguing: it will be interesting to see if other factors of this type exist, and whether they function as SRE-specific or signaling pathway-specific regulators of SRE function. In particular, it will be important to obtain cDNA clones encoding both $p62^{TCF}$ and the other binding proteins that have been detected in SRE-binding assays. Ultimately, these studies should allow elucidation of the pathways by which growth factors regulate immediate-early gene expression.

References

Ammerer, G. (1989). Identification, purification and cloning of a polypeptide (PRTF/GRM) that binds to mating-specific promoter elements in yeast. *Genes Dev.* **4**, 299–312.

Boxer, L. M., Prywes, R., Roeder, R. G., and Kedes, L. (1989). The sarcomeric actin CArG-binding factor is indistinguishable from the c-*fos* serum response factor. *Mol. Cell. Biol.* **9**, 515–522.

Bravo, R. (1990). Genes induced during the G_0/G_1 transition in mouse fibroblasts. *Semin. Cancer Biol.* **1**, 37–46.

Chow, K.-L., and Schwartz, R. J. (1990). A combination of closely associated positive and negative promoter elements regulates transcription of the skeletal α actin gene. *Mol. Cell. Biol.* **10**, 528–538.

Christy, B., and Nathans, D. (1989). Functional serum response elements upstream of the growth factor-inducible zif268. *Mol. Cell. Biol.* **9**, 4889–4895.

Dubois, E., Bercy, J., Descamps, F., and Messenguy, F. (1987). Characterisation of two new genes essential for vegetative growth of *Saccharomyces cerevisiae:* Nucleotide sequence determination and chromosome mapping. *Gene* **55**, 265–275.

Frederickson, R. M., Micheau, M. R., Iwamoto, A., and Miyamoto, N. G. (1989). 5′ flanking and first intron sequences of the human β actin gene required for efficient promoter activity. *Nucleic Acids Res.* **17**, 253–270.

Fujii, K., Sassone-Corsi, P., and Verma, I. M. (1988). c-*fos* promoter transactivation by the tax1 protein of human T-cell leukemia virus type 1. *Proc. Natl. Acad. Sci. U.S.A.* **85**, 8526–8530.

Gauthier-Rouviere, C., Fernandez, A., and Lamb, N. J. C. (1990). *ras*-Induced c-*fos* expression and proliferation in living rat fibroblasts involves C-kinase activation and the serum response element pathway. *EMBO J.* **9**, 171–180.

Gilman, M. Z., Wilson, R. N., and Weinberg, R. A. (1986). Multiple protein binding sites in the 5′ flanking region regulate c-*fos* expression. *Mol. Cell. Biol.* **6**, 4305–4314.

Gilman, M. Z. (1988). The c-*fos* SRE responds to protein kinase C-dependent and -independent signals but not to cyclic AMP. *Genes Dev.* **2**, 394–402.

Gius, D., Cao, X., Rauscher, F. J., III, Cohen, D. R., Curran, T., and Sukhatme, V. P. (1990). Transcriptional activation and repression by Fos are independent functions: The C-terminus represses immediate-early gene expression via CArG elements. *Mol. Cell. Biol.* **10**, 4243–4255.

Graham, R., and Gilman, M. Z. (1991). Distinct protein targets for signals acting at the c-fos serum response element. *Science* **251**, 189–192.

Greenberg, M. E., Siegfried, Z., and Ziff, E. B. (1987). Mutation of the c-*fos* dyad symmetry element inhibits inducibility *in vivo* and the nuclear regulatory factor binding *in vitro*. *Mol. Cell. Biol.* **7**, 1217–1225.

Gustafson, T. A., Taylor, A., and Kedes, L. (1989). DNA bending is induced by a transcription factor that interacts with the human c-*fos* and α-actin promoters. *Proc. Natl. Acad. Sci. U.S.A.* **86,** 2162–2166.

Hayes, T. E., Sengupta, P., and Cochran, B. H. (1988). The human serum response factor and the yeast factors GRM/PRTF have related DNA-binding specificities. *Genes Dev.* **2,** 1713–1722.

Herrera, R. E., Shaw, P. E., and Nordheim, A. (1989). Occupation of the c-*fos* serum response element *in vivo* by a multiprotein complex is unaltered by growth factor induction. *Nature* **340,** 68–70.

Herskowitz, I. (1989). A regulatory hierarchy for cell specialization in yeast. *Nature* **342,** 749–757.

Holt, J. T., Venkat-Gophal, T., Moulton, A. D., and Nienhuis, A. (1986). Inducible production of c-*fos* antisense RNA inhibits 3T3 cell proliferation. *Proc. Natl. Acad. Sci. U.S.A.* **83,** 4794–4798.

Jamal, S., and Ziff, E. B. (1990). Transactivation of c-*fos* and β actin genes by *raf* as a step in the early response to transmembrane signals. *Nature* **344,** 463–466.

Kaibuchi, K., Fukumoto, Y., Oku, N., Hori, Y., Yamamoto, T., Toyoshima, K., and Takai, Y. (1989). Activation of the serum response element and 12-O-tetradecanoylphorbol-13-acetate response element by the activated c-*raf*-1 protein in a manner independent of protein kinase C. *J. Biol. Chem.* **264,** 20855–20858.

Konig, H., Ponta, H., Rahmsdorf, U., Buscher, M., Schontal, A., Rahmsdorf, H. J., and Herrlich, P. (1989). Autoregulation of Fos: The dyad symmetry element as the major target of repression. *EMBO J.* **8,** 2559–2566.

Leung, S., and Miyamoto, N. G. (1989). Point mutational analysis of the human c-fos serum reponse factor binding site. *Nucleic Acids Res.* **17,** 1177–1195.

Levi, B-Z., Kasik, J. W., Burke, P. A., Prywes, R., Roeder, R. G., Appella, E., and Ozato, K. (1989). Neonatal induction of a protein that binds to the c-*fos* enhancer. *Proc. Natl. Acad. Sci. U.S.A.* **86,** 2262–2266.

Lucibello, F., Lowag, C., Neuberg, M., and Muller, R. (1989). Trans-repression of the mouse c-*fos* promoter: A novel mechanism of Fos-mediated trans-regulation. *Cell* **59,** 999–1007.

Luscher, B., Christenson, E., Litchfield, D. W., Krebs, E. G., and Eisenman, R. N. (1990). *Myb* DNA binding inhibited by phosphorylation at a site deleted during oncogenic activation. *Nature* **344,** 517–522.

Manak, J. R., de Bisschop, N., Kris, R. M., and Prywes, R. (1990). Casein kinase II enhances the DNA-binding activity of serum response factor. *Genes Dev.* **4,** 955–967.

Marais, R., Hsuan, J., McGuigan, C., Wynne, J., and Treisman, R. (1991). *EMBO J.*, manuscript submitted.

Minty, A., and Kedes, L. J. (1986). Upstream regions of the human cardiac actin gene that modulate its transcription in muscle cells: Presence of an evolutionarily conserved regulatory motif. *Mol. Cell. Biol.* **6,** 2125–2136.

Miwa, T., and Kedes, L. J. (1987). Duplicated CarG box domains have positive and mutually dependent regulatory roles in expression of the human α cardiac actin gene. *Mol. Cell. Biol.* **7,** 2803–2813.

Mohun, T. J., Garrett, N., and Treisman, R. H. (1987). *Xenopus* cytoskeletal actin and human c-*fos* gene promoters share a conserved protein binding site. *EMBO J.* **6**, 667–673.

Mohun, T. J., Taylor, M. J., Garrett, N., and Gurdon, J. B. (1989). The CArG promoter sequence is necessary for muscle-specific transcription of the cardiac actin gene in *Xenopus* embryos. *EMBO J.* **8**, 1153–1161.

Mohun, T. J., Chambers, A. E., Towers, N., and Taylor, M. V. (1991). Expression of genes encoding the transcription factor SRF during early development of Xenopus laevis: identification of a CArG box-binding activity as SRF. *EMBO J.* **10**, 933–940.

Muscat, G. E. O., Gustafson, T. A., and Kedes, L. (1988). A common factor regulates skeletal and cardiac α actin gene transcription in muscle. *Mol. Cell. Biol.* **8**, 4120–4133.

Nishikura, K., and Murray, J. M. (1987). Antisense RNA of protooncogene c-*fos* blocks renewed growth of quiescent 3T3 cells. *Mol. Cell. Biol.* **7**, 639–649.

Norman, C., and Treisman, R. (1988). Analysis of serum response element (SRE) function *in vitro*. *Cold Spring Harbor Symp. Quant. Biol.* **53**, 719–726.

Norman, C., Runswick, M., Pollock, R. M., and Treisman, R. (1988). Isolation and characterisation of cDNA clones encoding SRF, a transcription factor that binds the c-*fos* serum response element. *Cell* **55**, 989–1003.

Passmore, S., Maine, G. T., Elble, R., Christ, C., and Tye, B. K. (1988). A *Saccharomyces cerevisiae* protein involved in plasmid maintenance is necessary for mating of MATa cells. *J. Mol. Biol.* **204**, 593–606.

Passmore, S., Elble, R., and Tye, B. K. (1989). A protein involved in minichromosome maintenance in yeast binds a transcriptional enhancer conserved in eukaryotes. *Genes Dev.* **3**, 921–935.

Phan-Dinh-Tuy, F., Tuil, F., Schweighoffer, G., Pinset, C., Kahn, A., and Minty, A. (1988). The CC.Ar.GG box, a protein binding site common to transcription-regulatory regions of the cardiac actin, c-*fos* and interleukin-2 receptor genes. *Eur. J. Biochem.* **173**, 507–515.

Pollock, R. M., and Treisman, R. (1990). A sensitive method for the determination of protein-DNA binding specificities. *Nucleic Acids Res.* **18**, 6197–6204.

Pollock, R. M., and Treisman, R. (1991). Human SRF-related proteins: DNA binding properties and potential regulatory targets. *Genes and Devt.,* in press.

Prywes, R., and Roeder, R. G. (1986). Inducible binding of a factor to the c-*fos* enhancer. *Cell* **47**, 777–784.

Prywes, R., and Roeder, R. G. (1987). Purification of the c-*fos* enhancer binding protein. *Mol. Cell. Biol.* **7**, 3482–3489.

Prywes, R., Dutta, A., Cromlish, J. A., and Roeder, R. G. (1988). Phosphorylation of serum response factor, a factor that binds to the serum response element of the c-*fos* enhancer. *Proc. Natl. Acad. Sci. U.S.A.* **85**, 7206–7210.

Riabowol, K. T., Vosatka, R. J., Ziff, E. B., Lamb, N. J., and Feramisco, J. R. (1988). Microinjection of *fos*-specific antibodies blocks DNA synthesis in fibroblast cells. *Mol. Cell. Biol.* **8**, 1670–1677.

Rivera, V. M., and Greenberg, M. E. (1990). Growth factor-induced gene expression: The ups and downs of c-*fos* regulation. *New Biologist* **2**, 751–758.

Rivera, V. M., Sheng, M., and Greenberg, M. E. (1990). The inner core of the serum response element mediates both the rapid transcriptional induction and subsequent repression of c-*fos* transcription following serum stimulation. *Genes Dev.* **4,** 255–268.

Ryan, W. R., Jr., Franza, B. R., Jr., and Gilman, M. Z. (1989). Two distinct phosphoproteins bind to the c-*fos* serum response element. *EMBO J.* **8,** 1785–1792.

Sassonne-Corsi, P., Sisson, J. C., and Verma, I. M. (1988). Transcriptional autoregulation of the c-*fos* protooncogene. *Nature* **334,** 314–319.

Sassonne-Corsi, P., Der, C. D., and Verma, I. M. (1989). *ras*-Induced neuronal differentiation of PC-12 cells: Possible involvement of *fos* and *jun*. *Mol. Cell. Biol.* **9,** 3174–3183.

Schalasta, G., and Doppler, C. (1990). Inhibition of c-*fos* transcription and phosphorylation of the serum response factor by an inhibitor of phospholipase C-type reactions. *Mol. Cell. Biol.* **10,** 5558–5561.

Schonthal, A., Buscher, M., Angel, P., Rahmsdorf, H-J., Ponta, H., Hattori, K., Chiu, R., Karin, M., and Herrlich, P. (1989). The Fos and Jun/AP1 proteins are involved in the down-regulation of c-*fos* transcription. *Oncogene* **4,** 629–636.

Schroter, H., Shaw, P. E., and Nordheim, A. (1987). Purification of intercalator-released p67, a polypeptide that interacts specifically with the c-*fos* serum response element. *Nucleic Acids Res.* **15,** 10145–10158.

Schroter, H., Mueller, G. F., Meese, K., and Nordheim, A. (1990). Synergism in ternary complex formation between the dimeric glycoprotein p67/SRF, polypeptide p62/TCF, and the c-*fos* serum response element. *EMBO J.* **9,** 1123–1130.

Shaw, P. E., Schroter, H., and Nordheim, A. (1989a). The ability of a ternary complex to form over the serum response element correlates with serum inducibility of the c-*fos* promoter. *Cell* **56,** 563–572.

Shaw, P. E., Frasch, S., and Nordheim, A. (1989b). Repression of c-*fos* transcription is mediated through p67SRF bound to the SRE. *EMBO J.* **8,** 2567–2574.

Siegfried, Z., and Ziff, E. B. (1990). Altered transcriptional activity of c-*fos* promoter plasmids in V-*raf* transformed NIH 3T3 cells. *Mol. Cell. Biol.* **10,** 6073–6078.

Sommer, H., Beltran, J-P., Huiser, P., Pape, H., Lonnig, W-E., Saedler, H., and Schwarz-Sommer, Z. (1990). Deficiens, a homeotic gene involved in the control of flower morphogenesis in *Antirrhinum majus:* The protein shows homology to transcription factors. *EMBO J.* **9,** 605–613.

Sommercorn, J., Mulligan, J. A., Lozeman, F. J., and Krebs, E. J. (1987). Activation of casein kinase II in response to insulin and epidermal growth factor. *Proc. Natl. Acad. Sci. U.S.A.* **84,** 8834–8838.

Subramaniam, M., Schmidt, L. J., Crutchfield, C. E., III, and Getz, M. J. (1989). Negative regulation of serum-responsive enhancer elements. *Nature* **340,** 64–66.

Tan, S., and Richmond, T. J. (1990). DNA binding-induced conformational change of the yeast transcription activator PRTF. *Cell* **62,** 367–377.

Taylor, M. J., Treisman, R., Garrett, N., and Mohun, T. J. (1989). Muscle-specific (CArG) and serum-responsive (SRE) promoter elements are functionally interchangeable and bind serum response factor *in vitro*. *Development* **106,** 67–78.

Treisman, R. (1985). Transient accumulation of c-*fos* RNA following serum stimulation requires a conserved 5′ element and c-*fos* 3′ sequences. *Cell* **42,** 889–902.

Treisman, R. (1986). Identification of a protein-binding site that mediates transcription response of the c-*fos* gene to serum factors. *Cell* **46,** 567–574.

Treisman, R. (1987). Identification and purification of a polypeptide that binds the c-*fos* serum response element. *EMBO J.* **6,** 2711–2717.

Treisman, R. (1990). The SRE: A growth factor-responsive transcriptional regulator. *Semin. Cancer Biol.* **1,** 47–58.

Tuil, D., Clergue, N., Monterras, D., Pinset, C., Kahn, A., and Phan-Dinh-Tuy, F. (1990). CCArGG boxes, cis-acting elements with a dual specificity. *J. Mol. Biol.* **213,** 677–686.

Walsh, K., and Schimmel, P. (1987). Two nuclear factors compete for the skeletal muscle actin promoter. *J. Biol. Chem.* **262,** 9429–9432.

Walsh, K., and Schimmel, P. (1988). DNA-binding site for two skeletal actin promoter factors is important for expression in muscle cells. *Mol. Cell. Biol.* **8,** 1800–1802.

Walsh, K. (1989). Cross-binding of factors to functionally different promoter elements in c-*fos* and skeletal actin genes. *Mol. Cell. Biol.* **9,** 2191–2201.

Wilson, T. C., and Treisman, R. (1988). Fos C-terminal mutations block down-regulation of c-*fos* transcription following serum stimulation. *EMBO J.* **7,** 4193–4202.

Yanofsky, M. F., Ma, H., Bowman, J. L., Drews, G. L., Feldmann, K. A., and Meyerowitz, E. M. (1990). The protein encoded by the Arabidopsis homeotic gene agamous resembles transcription factors. *Nature* **346,** 35–39.

11

The Mouse H19 Gene: Its Structure and Function in Mouse Development

SHIRLEY M. TILGHMAN*, MARY E. BRUNKOW†, CAMILYNN I. BRANNAN‡, CLAIRE DEES§, MARISSA S. BARTOLOMEI‖, AND KATHARINE PHILLIPS#

**Howard Hughes Medical Institute*
and Department of Molecular Biology
Princeton University
Princeton, New Jersery

†Division of Molecular and
Developmental Biology
Samuel Lunenfeld Research Institute
Mt. Sinai Hospital
Toronto, Canada

‡NCI-FCRDC (National Cancer Institute-
Frederick Cancer Research & Development Center)
ABL-Basic Research Program
Frederick, Maryland

§Duke University School of Medicine
Durham, North Carolina

‖Department Molecular Biology
Princeton University
Princeton, New Jersey

#Thomas Jefferson University
School of Medicine
Philadelphia, Pennsylvania

I. Introduction

The majority of eukaryotic genes that have been characterized were first isolated using a detailed knowledge of the RNA or protein products they encoded. The advent of differential cDNA screening procedures, in which the transcriptional behavior of an RNA, rather than its product, was the basis for its isolation, has led to the cloning of cDNAs for which function must be sought. One of the first instances of such a screen, for the T cell-receptor genes (Hedrick *et al.*, 1984), provided an elegant example of the power of this approach. A more recent success was the isolation of the skeletal muscle regulatory gene, *myoD*, which is activated upon the differentiation of muscle progenitor cells (Davis *et al.*, 1987). In both instances the investigators had predicted that the genes they sought would have a specific transcriptional pattern, and therefore would be differentially represented in two related cell types.

The mouse H19 gene has been isolated four separate times in differential cDNA screens. It was originally identified in a screen for cDNAs, which were regulated by the trans-acting negative regulator of the mouse α-fetoprotein (AFP) gene, *raf* (Pachnis *et al.*, 1984). Expressed at high levels in the fetal liver, AFP is transcriptionally repressed shortly after birth (Tilghman and Belayew, 1982). BALB/cJ mice, which carry a recessive mutant allele of the *raf* gene, display hereditary persistence of AFP mRNA in liver (Belayew and Tilghman, 1982; Olsson *et al.*, 1977). A fetal cDNA library was screened by differential hybridization for mRNAs that decline after birth, to ask whether the *raf* gene regulates other liver-specific mRNAs after birth. One cDNA fulfilled this criterion, and was named H19 to designate its position on a filter.

The gene has now been cloned three additional times, first by Davis *et al.* (1987) during the screen for myoblast-specific cDNAs, which resulted in the cloning of the *myoD* gene. Indeed H19 RNA is expressed at a very low level in the progenitor stem cell, C3H10T1/2, and activated upon its differentiation to myoblasts (Pachnis *et al.*, 1988). Second, two independent groups (Wiles, 1988; F. Poirier and P. Rigby, personal communication, 1991) have identified H19 as a cDNA that activates upon embryonal carcinoma and embryonic stem cell differentiation, respectively.

Differential hybridization screens tend to be biased in favor of abundant RNAs, and H19 is no exception. The RNA is, in fact, one of the most abundant RNAs in the developing mouse embryo. In the midgestation embryo it is expressed in a broad array of tissues of both endoderm and mesoderm origin, including fetal liver, gut, lung, kidney, and skeletal and cardiac muscle. It is silent, however, in the central nervous system (H. Kim, A. Tyner, and S. M. Tilghman, unpublished results, 1991). Its expression begins at the blastocyst stage, and continues throughout development until shortly after birth, when its levels decline in all tissues, with the exception of skeletal muscle (Pachnis *et al.*, 1984).

II. Structure of the H19 Gene in Mice and Humans

When the mouse H19 gene was characterized in detail, it was immediately apparent that it was not a conventional mRNA (Pachnis *et al.*, 1988). The 3.0-kb gene is organized into five exons (Fig. 1), the largest of which is exon 1. The four introns are uniformly small, between 53 and 82 bp in length. The most unusual characteristic, however, was the absence of an open reading frame (ORF) that spanned some or all of the exons. Protein synthesis terminators peppered all three hypothetical reading frames (Fig. 2). In fact, the largest ORF was contained entirely within the first exon, sufficient to encode a protein of only 14 kDa (see the arrow in Fig. 2). That ORF was preceded by four AUG protein synthesis-initiation codons, which completely inhibited its translation *in vitro*.

All efforts to identify a protein corresponding to that reading frame were unsuccessful. Antibodies raised to fusion protein derivatives of the ORF did not recognize any protein in a wide variety of cell types that were tested (C. I. Brannan, unpublished observations, 1990). Likewise when a β-galactosidase protein was fused in-frame with the

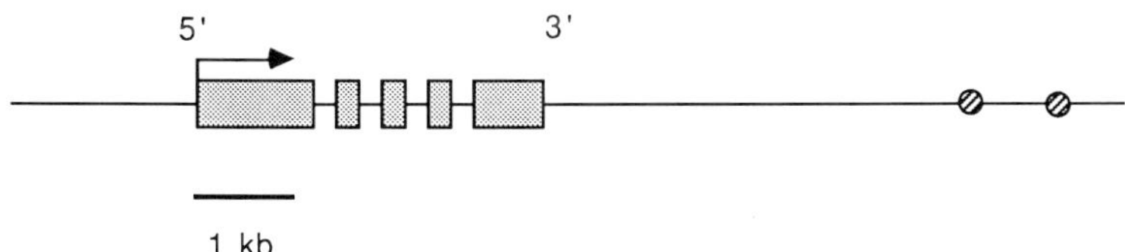

Fig. 1. The structure of the mouse H19 gene. The five exons of the mouse H19 gene are drawn as closed boxes, with the 5′ end of the gene marked by the arrow. The two 3′ distal enhancers are indicated by the hatched circles.

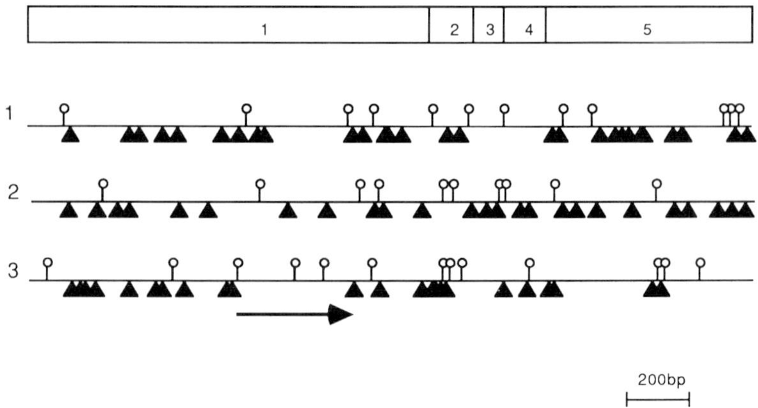

Fig. 2. The presence of open reading frames in the mouse H19 gene. The top line represents the 5 exons of the H19 cDNA. Lines 1–3 represent the three potential reading frames, marked with the positions of the AUG initiation codons (open circles) and protein synthesis termination codons (closed triangles). From Pachnis *et al.* (1988) and Brannan *et al.* (1990).

ORF and transfected into eukaryotic cells on an expression vector, no enzymatic or immunogenic β-galactosidase was detected.

These negative results raised the possibility that the mouse H19 gene was a pseudogene whose protein-coding sequence had been lost, but whose transcriptional competence had been retained, presumably by chance. If this were the case, the gene should not be recognizable in any other species. To test this possibility, we cloned and sequenced the human homolog (Brannan *et al.*, 1990). In both sequence and structure, the human H19 gene resembled very closely its murine counterpart. At the nucleotide level, the two genes were 77% identical; however, this figure is somewhat misleading, as the relatedness is unevenly distributed throughout the genes. The first half of exon 1, for example, is approximately 65% conserved, while the last half is over 85% conserved.

When the two H19 sequences were analyzed for the presence of common ORFs, the surprising result was that not a single ORF was conserved between them (Brannan *et al.*, 1990). The human RNA contains almost as many terminators in all three reading frames as the mouse counterpart, with the largest ORF encoding a completely different protein from the largest ORF in the mouse gene. So despite their marked similarity at the nucleotide level, they cannot encode a common protein.

The high degree of relatedness of the two genes eliminated the possibility that the H19 gene arose as a pseudogene before mammalian speciation. We cannot, however, exclude the possibility that it independently mutated in both mammalian species following speciation.

III. Structure and Localization of the H19 RNA

If the H19 gene does not encode a protein, what is the function of its abundant RNA product? Several possibilities are suggested by analyses of the structure of the RNA, its pattern of sequence conservation, and its intracellular localization.

By crude cell-fractionation studies, the RNA appeared to localize in the cytoplasmic rather than nuclear fraction of the cell. When cytoplasmic extracts of neonatal mouse liver were analyzed by sucrose gradient centrifugation, the RNA sedimented in a discrete 30S fraction (Fig. 3). This S value was significantly larger than that obtained with deproteinized RNA (bottom panel, Fig. 3), suggesting that the particle contained species other than H19 RNA. The behavior of the 30S particle was unaffected by the presence of ethylene diaminetetraacetic acid (EDTA), which disrupts the association between mRNAs and the ribosomes, as illustrated for the change in migration of albumin mRNA upon EDTA treatment. Indeed the analysis in Fig. 3 clearly illustrates that the H19 particle is not associated with ribosomes (Brannan *et al.*, 1990).

The sequestration of the H19 RNA into a cytoplasmic particle was not restricted to neonatal liver. Similar results were obtained in liver extracts obtained from animals at different stages of prenatal and postnatal development, in extracts derived from murine myoblast cell lines, and importantly, from extracts of human Hep3B cells. Thus the particle is not temporally, species- or tissue-specific.

RNA-folding computer programs predict that the RNA contains significant secondary structure, characteristic of RNAs such as snRNPs, rRNAs, and tRNAs. An examination of one of the most conserved domains of the RNA is instructive, both with respect to secondary structure and to the way in which the secondary structure is conserved between species. The area in question lies between nucleotides 994 and 1070 in the mouse RNA (hatched region in Fig. 4),

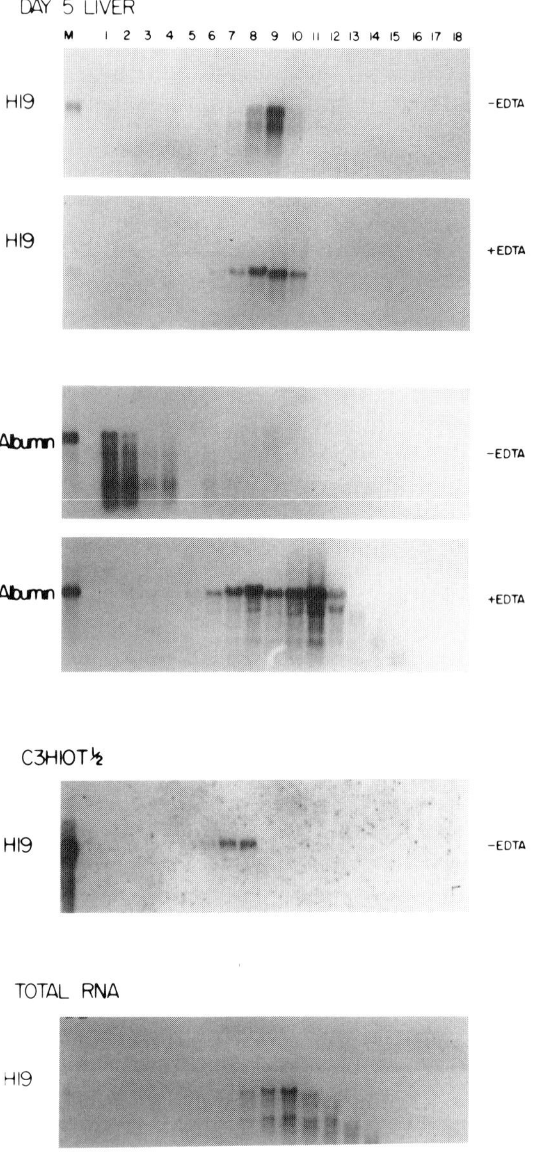

Fig. 3. The sedimentation of H19 RNA in a cytoplasmic particle. Postmitochondrial supernatants from day 5 livers or C3H 10T1/2 cells, untreated or incubated in the presence of EDTA, were sedimented in 10 to 40% sucrose gradients. Fractions were collected and analyzed for the presence of H19 RNA or albumin mRNA by Northern blot analysis. 28S rRNA migrates in fraction 10 of the gradient. The bottom of the tube is to the left. The bottom panel represents the migration of deproteinized H19 RNA. From Brannan *et al.* (1990).

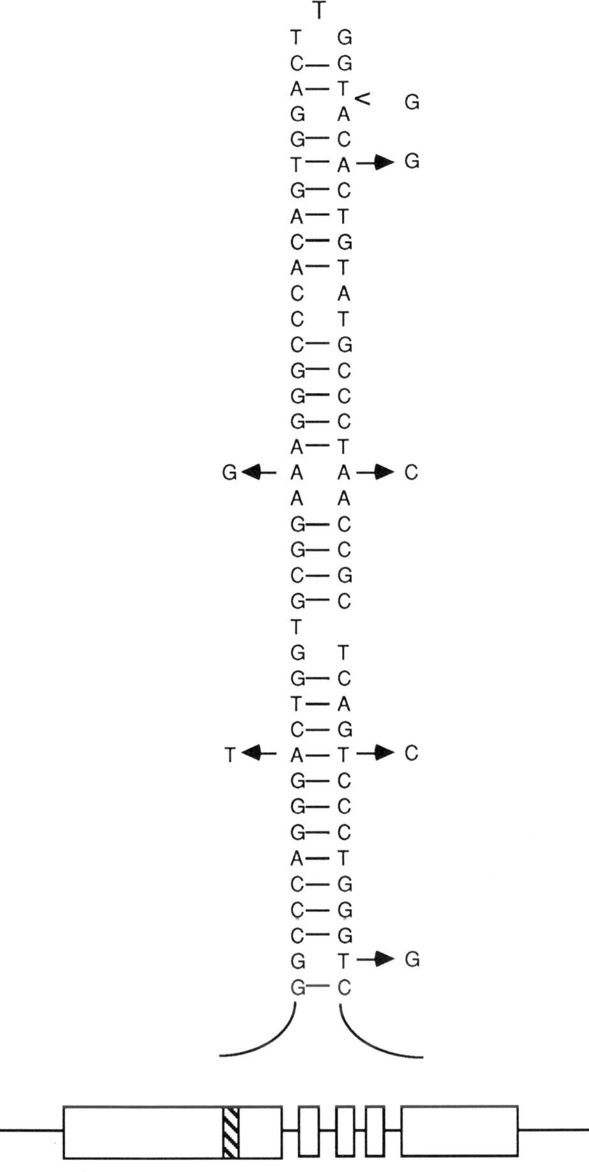

Fig. 4. The presence and conservation of secondary structure in H19 RNA. A segment of the mouse H19 RNA, taken from the hatched box in the gene diagram (below) is drawn as an extended inverted repeat. The arrows indicate positions where the human and mouse RNA sequences differ.

and it can be drawn as a long inverted repeat. If we examine the bases within this region that are different in the human RNA, indicated in Fig. 4 by the arrows, four of the seven fall within complementary base pairs. These four changes do not alter the overall number of complementary base pairs within the inverted repeat, as the human gains one base pair and loses one, relative to the mouse RNA. Of the other three changes, two are close to the loop of the inverted repeat, and one lies at its base and does not add to or decrease a base pair. This pattern of conservation suggests that the RNA's structure is important and subject to evolutionary pressure.

As was indicated earlier, the degree of sequence conservation of the H19 RNA between humans and mice is not uniform, but varies considerably from one part of the RNA to another. This punctate pattern is reminiscent of RNAs that function within RNA–protein complexes. For example the RNA moiety essential for the telomerase enzymatic activity in ciliated protozoa is not well conserved across protozoan species, except for the segments that are essential to its priming function (Shippen-Lentz and Blackburn, 1990). Likewise the RNA subunit of RNase P is not well conserved in either prokaryotes (Gold and Altman, 1986; Reed, 1984) or yeast (Lee and Engelke, 1989). Finally the demonstration that the trans-spliced leaders of *Caenorhabditis elegans* and trypanosomes share a conserved secondary structure with U1 RNA that they functionally replace, illustrates the importance of secondary structure in the function of these classes of RNAs (Bruzik *et al.*, 1988).

Thus in terms of structure and localization in a particle, the H19 RNA most closely resembles RNAs that function within the cell as part of RNA–protein complexes. These complexes carry out diverse sets of enzymatic reactions, from nuclear RNA processing in the case of the snRNPs (Maniatis and Reed, 1987), protein targeting, in the case of the signal recognition particle (Walter and Blobel, 1982), to telomere synthesis (Greider and Blackburn, 1987). H19 RNA differs from these examples in one very important respect, however, in that it is not ubiquitously expressed in mammals. Its restricted tissue specificity and repression after birth indicate that it cannot carry out a function necessary for all cells. Rather its function must be one that is necessary during development, but may be dispensed with in most tissues after birth.

The cytoplasmic localization would suggest that neither transcription, nuclear processing, nor transport into the cytoplasm is involved in H19 gene function. This conclusion must be tempered, however, until a more rigorous demonstration of intracellular localization by RNA *in situ* hybridization or immunocytochemistry is performed. There are several instances in which RNAs with nuclear function fractionate biochemically into the cytoplasm.

Two other RNA polymerase II products that do not apparently encode a functional protein have been described recently. The *hsr omega* gene in *Drosophila melanogaster,* originally identified because of its response to heat shock, is thought to function as a translational regulator (Fini *et al.,* 1989). An antisense RNA in *Xenopus laevis* may regulate the concentration of fibroblast growth factor mRNA (Kimelman and Kirschner, 1989). Neither example is consistent with our observations regarding H19 RNA, as we cannot detect its presence associated with the translation machinery, and no sense transcript has been detected to date.

IV. Transcriptional Control of the Murine H19 Gene

In addition to its unusual properties, the H19 gene displays a complex pattern of gene expression in the mouse. It is activated early in development in the blastocyst, maintained at high levels in cells of both endoderm and mesoderm, and repressed after birth in all but skeletal muscle derivatives. We could imagine at one extreme a model whereby this complex pattern is determined by a large number of regulatory regions, one for each specific pattern. The other extreme would have the gene regulated by a single control region more closely resembling that of a constitutively expressed gene. Resolving this issue requires a complete understanding of the elements that contribute to its complex pattern of expression.

Toward that end, modified copies of the H19 gene were introduced by transfection into a human hepatoma cell line, Hep3B, which expresses the human gene (Yoo-Warren *et al.,* 1988). The gene itself was used, rather than a reporter gene, because of the possibility that regulatory elements existed within the gene itself. These experiments identified three regions that appeared to contribute to high-level expression of the gene within liver cells: a promoter-proximal domain of approximately 130 bp, and two 3′ distal enhancers that lay 8 and 9.5 kb 3′ of the transcriptional start site (Fig. 1). Not surprisingly, these enhancers displayed motifs that were also present in the enhancers of the AFP gene (Godbout *et al.*, 1988; Yoo-Warren *et al.*, 1988).

The same constructs were introduced into PC13 cells, an embryonal carcinoma cell line that can be induced to differentiate into visceral endoderm, to ask whether the liver-specific enhancers also functioned in another endoderm lineage. Activation of the transfected H19 gene could be demonstrated in these cells, and that activation was dependent on the presence of the two 3′ distal enhancers (Yoo-Warren *et al.*, 1988). Thus at least two cell types appear to utilize the same transcriptional elements to achieve gene activation.

At this time nothing is known about the elements that control the mesoderm expression of the H19 gene. Neither of the liver-specific enhancers displays any activity by transfection in myoblast cell lines that are expressing the endogenous gene at high levels (M. Brunkow, unpublished observations, 1990). In two other respects, the muscle and liver appear to regulate the gene using different mechanisms. The expression of the H19 gene in skeletal muscle is not affected by alleles of the *raf* gene that alter the adult basal level of H19 RNA in liver (Pachnis *et al.*, 1984). The gene also responds to growth arrest differently in the two tissues, in that its expression is positively correlated with cell division in liver (Pachnis *et al.*, 1984), whereas it is activated in C3H10T1/2 cells upon growth arrest (Pachnis *et al.*, 1988).

V. Genetic Analysis of the Murine H19 Gene

The mouse H19 gene has been mapped to the distal end of mouse chromosome 7, together with the insulin growth factor II, insulin-2, tyrosine hydroxylase, and *int*-2 genes (Pachnis *et al.*, 1984; T. Glaser and D. Housman, personal communication, 1991). This region of the mouse genome has been identified by Cattanach (Cattanach, 1986) as a region that undergoes genomic imprinting. That is, either maternal duplication/paternal deficiency or paternal duplication/maternal deficiency generated by nondisjunction in intercrosses between animals harboring balanced translocations involving chromosome 7 results in prenatal lethality (see Solter, 1988). This presumably means that there are genes in this region whose overexpression or underexpression is deleterious to mice.

The repression of the H19 gene in liver after birth is mediated at least in part by a substantial decrease in its rate of transcription, based on nuclear run-on analysis (C. I. Brannan, unpublished observations, 1990). It is also influenced by at least two unlinked loci: *raf*, which determines in part its adult basal level and *Rif*, which determines its degree of inducibility during liver regeneration (Pachnis *et al.*, 1984). Only one mutant allele of the *raf* gene, which is located on the proximal portion of chromosome 15 roughly midway between c-*myc* and an α-globin pseudogene-3 (Blankenhorn *et al.*, 1988; S. Tilghman, unpublished observations, 1990) has been described (Olsson *et al.*, 1977). In BALB/cJ mice, the levels of H19 RNA are 20- to 50-fold higher in adult liver than in any other inbred or wild mouse strains tested (Pachnis *et al.*, 1984), although the mechanism underlying this elevation has not been determined.

The *Rif* gene has not been mapped in the mouse, and either heterozygotes or homozygotes carrying the dominant *Rif-b* allele found in C57BL/6J mice display a limited inducibility of H19 during liver regeneration, as compared to other inbred strains. Both loci also affect AFP expression in the same manner, indicating that the mechanisms regulating these genes, at least in liver, are probably similar.

VI. Summary

The H19 gene has been cloned multiple times because of its relative abundance in differentiated cells. The absence of an ORF and the localization of the RNA to a cytoplasmic particle are consistent with the RNA functioning as an RNA, either alone or together with proteins. Its conservation in mammals suggests that it is under selective pressure in evolution, and likely to be of functional importance to the embryo. Two paths are available to probe the nature of that function. The biochemical identification of the constituents of the RNP particle will be essential to understanding the particle's function. Alternatively, mutations in mice that result in both gain-of-function and loss-of-function phenotypes should help to establish the role of this RNA in development.

References

Belayew, A., and Tilghman, S. M. (1982). Genetic analysis of α-fetoprotein synthesis in mice. *Mol. Cell. Biol.* **2**, 1427–1435.

Blankenhorn, E. P., Duncan, R., Huppi, K., and Potter, M. (1988). Chromosomal location of the regulator of mouse α-fetoprotein, Afr-1. *Genetics* **119**, 687–691.

Brannan, C. I., Dees, E. C., Ingram, R. S., and Tilghman, S. M. (1990). The product of the H19 gene may function as an RNA. *Mol. Cell. Biol.* **10**, 28–36.

Bruzik, J. P., Van Doren, K., Hirsh, D., and Steitz, J. A. (1988). Trans-splicing involves a novel form of small nuclear ribonucleoprotein particles. *Nature (London)* **335**, 559–562.

Cattanach, B. M. (1986). Parental origin effects in mice. *J. embrol. exp. Morph.* (Suppl.) **97**, 137–150.

Davis, R. L., Weintraub, H., and Lassar, A. B. (1987). Expression of a single transfected cDNA converts fibroblasts to myoblasts. *Cell* **51**, 987–1000.

Fini, M. E., Bendena, W. G., and Pardue, M. L. (1989). Unusual behavior of the cytoplasmic transcript of *hsr omega:* An abundant, stress-inducible RNA that is translated but yields no detectable protein product. *J. Cell Biol.* **108**, 2045–2057.

Godbout, R., Ingram, R. S., and Tilghman, S. M. (1988). Fine-structure mapping of the three mouse α-fetoprotein gene enhancers. *Mol. Cell. Biol.* **8**, 1169–1178.

Gold, H. A., and Altman, S. (1986). Reconstitution of RNAse P activity using inactive subunits from *E. coli* and HeLa cells. *Cell* **44**, 243–249.

Greider, C. W., and Blackburn, E. H. (1987). The telomere terminal transferase of Tetrahymena is a ribonucleoprotein enzyme with two kinds of primer specificity. *Cell* **51**, 887–898.

Hedrick, S. M., Cohen, D. I., Nielsen, E. A., and Davis, M. M. (1984). Isolation of cDNA clones encoding T cell-specific membrane-associated proteins. *Nature (London)* **308**, 149–153.

Kimelman, D., and Kirschner, M. W. (1989). An antisense mRNA directs the covalent modification of the transcript encoding fibroblast growth factor in *Xenopus* oocytes. *Cell* **59**, 697–696.

Lee, J.-Y., and Engelke, D. R. (1989). Partial characterization of an RNA component that copurifies with *Saccharomyces cerevisiae* RNAse P. *Mol. Cell. Biol.* **9**, 2536–2543.

Maniatis, T., and Reed, R. (1987). The role of small nuclear ribonucleoprotein particles in pre-mRNA splicing. *Nature (London)* **325**, 673–678.

Olsson, M., Lindahl, G., and Ruoshahti, E. (1977). Genetic control of alpha-fetoprotein synthesis in the mouse. *J. Exp. Med.* **145**, 819–827.

Pachnis, V., Belayew, A., and Tilghman, S. M. (1984). Locus unlinked to α-fetoprotein under the control of the murine *raf* and *Rif* genes. *Proc. Natl. Acad. Sci. U.S.A.* **81**, 5523–5527.

Pachnis, V., Brannan, C. I., and Tilghman, S. M. (1988). The structure and expression of a novel gene activated in early mouse embryogenesis. *EMBO J.* **7**, 673–681.

Reed, R. E. (1984). "A Study of the RNA Component of *E. coli* RNAse P." Ph.D. Thesis, Yale University, New Haven, Connecticut.

Shippen-Lentz, D., and Blackburn, E. H. (1990). Functional evidence for an RNA template in telomerase. *Science* **247**, 546–552.

Solter, D. (1988). Differential imprinting and expression of maternal and paternal genomes. *Annu. Rev. Genet.* **22**, 127–146.

Tilghman, S. M., and Belayew, A. (1982). Transcriptional control of the murine albumin/alpha-fetoprotein locus during development. *Proc. Natl. Acad. Sci. U.S.A.* **79**, 5254–5257.

Walter, P., and Blobel, G. (1982). Signal-recognition particle contains a 7S RNA essential for protein translocation across the endoplasmic reticulum. *Nature (London)* **299**, 691–698.

Wiles, M. V. (1988). Isolation of differentially expressed human cDNA clones: Similarities between mouse and human embryonal carcinoma cell differentiation. *Development* **104**, 403–413.

Yoo-Warren, H., Pachnis, V., Ingram, R. S., and Tilghman, S. M. (1988). Two regulatory domains flank the mouse H19 gene. *Mol. Cell. Biol.* **8**, 4707–4715.

12

Regulation of Transcription in Animal Cells: Factors and Mechanisms

B. Franklin Pugh[1] AND Robert Tjian

Howard Hughes Medical Institute
Department of Molecular and Cell Biology
University of California, Berkeley
Berkeley, California

I. Introduction

The synthesis of mRNA is a critical control point in the differential regulation of gene expression in mammalian cells. A wealth of studies in the past 10 years have established that a particular class of nuclear

[1]*Present address:* Department of Molecular and Cell Biology, The Pennsylvania State University, University Park, Pennsylvania 16802

proteins, the sequence-specific DNA-binding transcription factors are responsible, in large measure, for regulating the activity of genes by turning up or down the rate of transcriptional initiation.

This fascinating group of protein factors operate by recognizing and binding to selected sequences in the genome of an organism that are designated as promoter/enhancer regions. Once these regulatory factors are tethered to specific DNA sequences contained within promoter elements, they are able to activate or repress the basal level of transcription by mechanisms that still remain largely unknown. In addition to the action of promoter-selective enhancer factors, the rates of mRNA synthesis are also dependent on the concerted function of a complex assembly of proteins and enzymes commonly referred to as the transcription machinery, which includes RNA polymerase II and a variety of accessory factors that help catalyze the accurate and efficient initiation of transcription from promoter sequences (reviewed in Saltzman and Weinmann, 1989).

The purification and cloning of various genes that encode mammalian DNA-binding transcription factors, as well as some of the basal accessory factors of the general transcriptional apparatus, have provided the opportunity to analyze the structure, function, and mechanism by which these different classes of nuclear proteins interact to govern transcription and gene expression. Of particular interest is the finding that several transcription factors are encoded by protooncogenes and that the ability to cause neoplastic transformation and oncogenesis may be linked to the aberrant activity of altered transcription factors. Thus, the mechanism by which sequence-specific transcription factors regulate gene activity has become a central focus in our quest to understand not only nuclear processes but also oncogenesis.

II. Transcriptional Activation Pathways

The basal initiation complex consisting of RNA polymerase II and accessory factors can assemble and initiate specifically at a minimal promoter consisting of a TATA box and initiator DNA element (Saltzman and Weinmann, 1989). The TATA box binds the TBP (for TATA binding protein) subunit of the TFIID complex, which is thought to serve as a nucleating center for the subsequent assembly of the other basal factors including RNA polymerase II (Buratowski *et al.*, 1989; Horikoshi *et al.*, 1989; Peterson *et al.*, 1990). The role of sequence-specific transcription factors is apparently to enhance or repress the basal transcription capacity. Sequence-specific transcription factors have also been well established as a major determinant governing gene regulation and cellular differentiation, yet little is known about the molecular pathways that lead to promoter activation. For example, although DNA-binding and transcription activation domains of many trans-activators have been characterized structurally and functionally, the actual targets of these activators and their mode of action is not known. Similarly, RNA polymerase II and its accessory or basal initiation factors (TFIIA, -B, -D, -E, -F, and G) have been poorly characterized, and in some cases still remain as impure fractions. Consequently, the crucial interplay between basal factors and promoter-selective regulators remains to be unraveled.

III. Properties of Transcriptional Regulatory Proteins

Trans-activators are typically composed of modular units, including a domain for DNA binding and one or more for transcriptional activation (reviewed in Mitchell and Tjian, 1989). One particularly striking feature of many activation domains is the preponderance of one of the following classes of amino acids: glu/asp (acidic), gln, and pro (Mitchell and Tjian, 1989). Prototypic trans-activators of each class are GAL4, Sp1, and CTF, respectively. Except for *richness* in a particular amino acid, there is little sequence and, presumably, structural similarity among activation domains even within a class. Thus, there is scant reason to assume that they function by the same molecular mechanism. Thus far, the physiological targets for the various trans-activators have not been identified.

Candidates for trans-activator targets include components of chromatin, basal initiation factors, subunits of RNA polymerase II, and various intermediary factors including *coactivators, adaptors,* and *mediators,* which are hypothesized to transduce the signal from the trans-activator to the basal complex (Horikoshi *et al.*, 1988a; Horikoshi *et al.*, 1988b; Pugh and Tjian, 1990). One popular model proposes that some activation domains directly contact the TATA binding protein (TBP) to stabilize its binding at the promoter (Ptashne, 1988). Evidence indicates that the hybrid acidic activator

GAL4/VP16 can directly interact with cloned yeast TFIID stringer. However, no evidence has been obtained to demonstrate that TFIID/VP16 complexes represent active intermediates in the assembly of a preinitiation complex. Indeed, other reports suggest that the acidic activation domain of GAL4/VP16 acts primarily to derepress templates assembled into chromatin (Workman *et al.*, 1991; Croston *et al.*, 1991). The same acidic activation domain has also been implicated in functioning through adaptors or mediators, which in turn are proposed to contact the basal initiation complex (Berger *et al.* 1990; Kelleher *et al.*, 1990; Flanagan *et al.*, 1991). At present, we have not been able to determine which, if any or all, of these potential pathways is correct.

Activators might function at one level to alter chromatin composition or structure either directly, or by assisting the basal initiation factors and RNA polymerase II to gain access to the promoter DNA sequence. Once the chromatin-bound promoter has been derepressed and the preinitiation complex established, the trans-activator might facilitate the release of RNA polymerase II to transcribe the gene. The core histone subunits of chromatin need not be the only *generalized* transcriptional inhibitor that trans-activators must overcome. Other histone-like proteins might also contribute to the global repression of genes.

Thus, there might be multiple distinct mechanisms that lead to promoter activation, and any one might have variations on the same theme, which the cell can exploit. In addition, a trans-activator might utilize more than one mechanism, either by having multiple activation domains or by engaging a single domain in more than one step in the activation pathway.

IV. Activation by Sp1: A Glutamine-Rich Activator

To address these different potential mechanisms, we focused on the glutamine-rich activation domains of the human transcription factor Sp1. We first asked whether Sp1 activates transcription solely by derepressing the promoter from inhibitors. If Sp1 serves to remove global-type inhibitors, then the template should become more accessible to the basal initiation machinery, such as TFIID. In our Sp1-

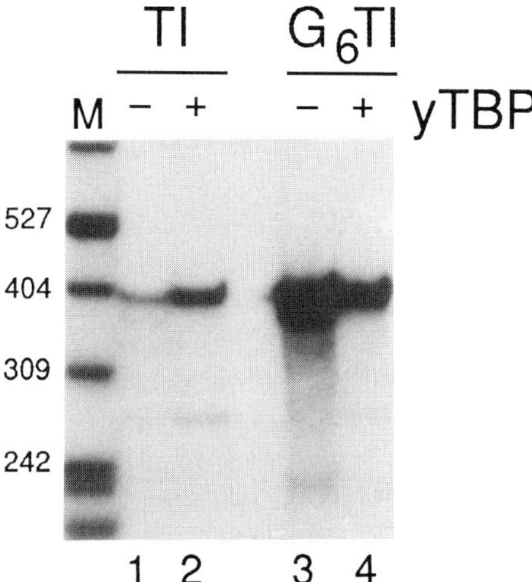

Fig. 1. Yeast TBP behaves dominantly over human TFIID. Transcription reactions were reconstituted with partially purified HeLa TFIIA, TFIIB, TFIIE/F pol II, TFIID, and purified Sp1 as described in Pugh and Tjian (1990). Lanes 1–2 contained TATA/Inr templates; lanes 3–4 contained TATA/Inr templates with 6 Sp1 binding sites upstream of the TATA box. Reactions in lanes 2 and 4 contained 30 ng of pure yeast TBP in addition to the basal factors listed above.

responsive reconstituted transcription reactions, the TFIID concentration is limiting and sets the observed level of basal transcription. As previously established (Buratowski *et al.*, 1988; Cavallini *et al.*, 1988), addition of purified cloned yeast TBP to a complete reaction, reconstituted on the minimal TATA/initiator promoter lacking Sp1 binding sites, results in increased levels of basal transcription (Fig. 1, lanes 1 and 2). However, addition of the yeast TBP to an Sp1-responsive human transcription reaction, containing the human TFIID complex, actually decreases the level of transcription (Fig. 1, lanes 3 and 4). Yeast TBP is therefore somehow incompatible with the ability of Sp1 to activate transcription and even dominantly interferes with the functioning of human TBP present in the TFIID complex. These observations are not consistent with the simple model that Sp1 merely serves to remove a nonspecific inhibitor to allow the general transcription machinery access to the promoter. Instead the data suggest that Sp1 might require the homologous human TBP to assemble a proper initiation complex, and that the yeast protein bears species-specific differences that preclude the formation of a productive Sp1-responsive complex.

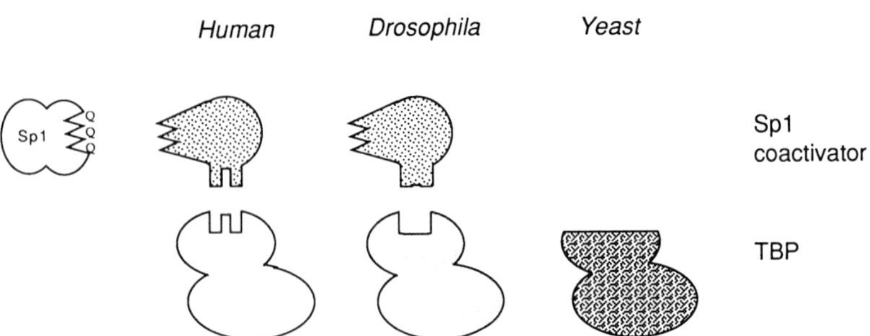

Fig. 2. A schematic of some of the regulatory factors involved in Sp1-activated transcription. Activities (coactivator and TBP) are illustrated in rows, whereas the proposed species specific difference are found in different columns. Yeast does not appear to have coactivators that allow Sp1 to activate transcription.

V. Structure and Function of Yeast, *Drosophila*, and Human TBP

We recently cloned cDNAs encoding *drosophila* and human TBP (Hoey *et al.*, 1990; Peterson *et al.*, 1990). A comparison of yeast, *drosophila*, and human TBP proteins reveals a striking bipartite structure with distinct functional domains. The C-terminal 180 amino acids of TBP is highly conserved and is sufficient to bind TATA boxes and interact with TFIIA and -B to promote basal transcription. In contrast, activation by Sp1 requires the nonconserved N-terminal portion of TBP. However, replacement of the partially purified HeLa TFIID fraction with the cloned human, *drosophila*, or yeast TBP protein in a transcription reaction reconstituted with fractionated HeLa initiation factors is not sufficient to restore an Sp1-response. Instead, Sp1 requires a coactivator that normally copurifies with human TBP and that we hypothesize functions as a molecular adaptor connecting the activation domain of Sp1 to the basal transcription apparatus through the amino-terminal portion of TBP (Pugh and Tjian, 1990). The activator/coactivator interface appears functionally conserved between species, whereas the coactivator/TBP interface appears to be species specific (Fig. 2).

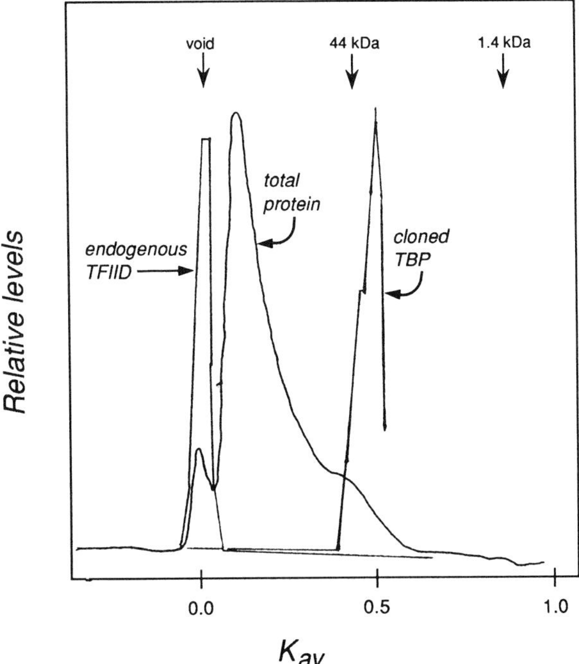

Fig. 3. Gel filtration chromatography of endogenous TFIID and cloned human TBP. A sephacryl S300HR column was loaded with partially purified HeLa TFIID as described in Pugh and Tjian (1990). Much of the total protein runs between 400 and 200 kDa, while the HeLa TFIID runs at >700 kDa. Recombinant human TBP overexpressed in HeLa cells was partially purified and applied to the column as described by Peterson *et al.* (1990). K_{av} is defined in Pugh and Tjian (1990) and represents the fraction of the column included volume.

VI. Human TBP Is in a TFIID Complex with the Sp1 Coactivator

Chromatography of the endogenous HeLa TFIID fraction over six different ion exchange and gel filtration columns failed to separate the Sp1 coactivator from the TFIID activity, suggesting that the coactivator might be tightly associated with TFIID. When cloned human TBP is overexpressed in HeLa cells, partially purified, and subjected to S-300 gel filtration chromatography, the recombinant protein migrates according to its predicted molecular mass of 38 kDa (Fig. 3).

However, when endogenous TFIID is chromatographed over the same column, it is excluded from the beads, indicating that the endogenous TFIID may reside in a relatively stable macromolecular complex of over 700 kDa. Western blot analysis of the TFIID polypeptide in this endogenous complex reveals that the TFIID is the same molecular mass as the cloned factor expressed in *Escherichia coli.* Consistent with the possibility that TFIID might be complexed with a number of different coactivators, the chromatographic properties of the endogenous TFIID activity is very heterogeneous, eluting over a broad salt range on phosphocellulose, DEAE-sepharose, FPLC mono Q, and mono S.

The interaction of different coactivators with TFIID might provide a means for the various classes of activation domains to interface with a common basal initiation factor. Not only is site-specific binding required for trans-activators to function, but their respective coactivator must also be present to complete the promoter circuitry. Thus, two trans-activators such as Oct 1 and Oct 2, which bind the same sequence, may be present in the same cell type yet have differential activating potential.

VII. Negative Regulation of the Protooncogene Jun

Whereas coactivators provide a means for stimulating transcription initiation, some may function negatively, perhaps by binding to the activation domain but not allowing productive interactions with TFIID. Evidence for such negative regulators has recently been found for the proto-oncoprotein c-jun.

Analysis of transcriptional activation properties of c-jun in different cell lines by transient transfection experiments suggests that it contains an activator domain (A1) that is negatively regulated by a cell-type specific inhibitor (Baichwal and Tjian, 1990). These experiments also reveal that a regulatory domain of c-jun, δ, previously identified by *in vitro* experiments, also regulates transcriptional activation by c-jun *in vivo*. The δ domain facilitates or stabilizes the interaction of the cellular inhibitor with A1. Although it lacks δ, v-jun is a stronger transcriptional activator than c-jun, both *in vivo* and *in vitro,* since its activity is not efficiently repressed by the cellular inhibitor. *In vitro* transcription experiments with chimeric jun proteins and extracts from different cell types confirm that the activity of the A1 and δ domains is cell-type specific. These findings implicate a specific cellular factor in the negative regulation of c-jun transcriptional activity and suggest a molecular basis for the observed difference in transcriptional activity between v-jun and c-jun.

The involvement of coactivators in the trans-activation process may be only one segment in the entire gene-activation pathway. Additional possibly direct interactions of trans-activators with chromatin and the basal initiation factors would contribute substantially to tight regulatory control of the promoter.

References

Baichwal, V. W., and Tjian, R. (1990). Control of c-jun activity by interaction of a cell-specific inhibitor with regulatory domain δ: differences between v- and c-jun. *Cell* **63,** 815–825.

Berger, S. L., Cress, W. D., Cress, A., Triezenberg, S. J., and Guarente, L. (1990). Selective inhibition of activated but not basal transcription by the acidic activation domain of VP16: evidence for transcriptional adaptors. *Cell* **61,** 1199–1208.

Buratowski, S., Hahn, S., Guarente, L., and Sharp, P. A. (1989). Five intermediate complexes in transcription initiation by RNA polymerase II. *Cell* **56,** 549–561.

Buratowski, S., Hahn, S., and Sharp, A. (1988). Function of a yeast TATA element binding protein in a mammalian transcription system. *Nature (London)* **334,** 37–42.

Cavallini, B., Huet, J., Plassat, J., Sentenac, A., Egly, J., and Chambon, P. (1988). A yeast activity can substitute for the HeLa cell TATA box factor. *Nature (London)* **334,** 77–80.

Croston, G. E., Kerrigan, L. A., Lira, L. M., Marshak, D. R., and Kadonaga, J. T. (1991). Sequence-specific antirepression of histone H1-mediated inhibition of basal RNA polymerase II transcription. *Science* **251,** 643–649.

Flanagan, P. M., Kelleher, R. J., III, Sayre, M. H., Tschochner, H., and Kornberg, R. D. (1991). A mediator required for activation of RNA polymerase II transcription in vitro. *Nature (London)* **350,** 436–438.

Hoey, T., Dynlacht, B. D., Peterson, M. G., Pugh, B. F., and Tjian, R. (1990). Isolation and characterization of the Drosophila gene encoding the TATA binding protein, TFIID. *Cell* **61,** 1179–1186.

Horikoshi, M., Carey, M. F., Kakidani, H., and Roeder, R. G. (1988a). Mechanism of action of a yeast activator: Direct effect of Gal4 derivatives on mammalian TFIID-promoter interactions. *Cell* **54,** 665–669.

Horikoshi, M., Hai, T., Lin, Y.-S., Green, M. R., and Roeder, R. G. (1988b). Transcription factor ATF interacts with the TATA factor to facilitate establishment of a preinitiation complex. *Cell* **54,** 1033–1042.

Horikoshi, M., Wang, C. K., Fujii, H., Cromlish, J. A., Weil, P. A., and Roeder, R. G.

(1989). Purification of a yeast TATA box-binding protein that exhibits human transcription factor IID activity. *Proc. Natl. Acad. Sci. U.S.A.* **86,** 4843–4847.

Kelleher, R. J., III, Flanagan, P. M., and Kornberg, R. D. (1990). A novel mediator between activator proteins and the RNA polymerase II transcription apparatus. *Cell* **61,** 1209–1215.

Mitchell, P. J., and Tjian, R. (1989). Transcriptional regulation in mammalian cells by sequence-specific DNA-binding proteins. *Science* **245,** 371–378.

Peterson, M. G., Tanese, N., Pugh, B. F., and Tjian, R. (1990). Functional domains and upstream activation properties of cloned human TATA binding protein. *Science* **248,** 1625–1630.

Ptashne, M. (1988). How eukaryotic transcriptional activators work. *Nature (London)* **335,** 683–689.

Pugh, B. F., and Tjian, R. (1990). Mechanism of transcriptional activation by Sp1: Evidence for coactivators. *Cell* **61,** 1187–1197.

Saltzman, A. G., and Weinmann, R. (1989). Promoter specificity and modulation of RNA polymerase II transcription. *FASEB J.* **3,** 1723–1733.

Workman, J. L., Taylor, I. C. A., and Kingston, R. E. (1991). Activation domains of stably bound GAL4 derivatives alleviate repression of promoters by nucleosomes. *Cell* **64,** 533–544.

Index

S

T

BRISTOL-MYERS SQUIBB CANCER SYMPOSIA

10. Emil Frei III (Editor).
The Regulation of Proliferation and Differentiation in Normal and Neoplastic Cells, 1989.

11. Roswell K. Boutwell and Ilse L. Riegel (Editors).
The Cellular and Molecular Biology of Human Carcinogenesis, 1989.

12. Baniel E. Bergsagel and Tak W. Mak (Editors).
Molecular Mechanisms and Their Clinical Application in Malignancies, 1991.

13. Takashi Tsuruo and Makoto Ogawa (Editors).
Drug Resistance as a Biochemical Target in Cancer Chemotherapy, 1991.

14. Phillip A. Sharp (Editor).
Nuclear Processes and Oncogenes, 1992.